Coping

Stress and the Major Cardiovascular Disorders

ROBERT S. ELIOT, M.D., F.A.C.C.

Professor of Medicine

*Monsour Medical Foundation Professor
of Cardiovascular Medicine*

*Director of the Cardiovascular Center
and the Division of Cardiovascular Medicine*

*The University of Nebraska Medical Center
Omaha, Nebraska*

FUTURA PUBLISHING COMPANY
Mount Kisco, New York
1979

Copyright © 1979
Futura Publishing Company

Published by
Futura Publishing Company
295 Main Street
Mount Kisco, New York 10549

LC: 79-50814
ISBN: 0-87993-120-5

Typography by Topel Typographic Corp., New York City

*In memory of Doctor Paul H. Burgert,
whose life and practice portrayed the principles
pursued in this text.*

*This book is dedicated to those who strive
to balance the science and technology
with the art of medicine.*

CONTENTS

INTRODUCTION

We are frequently struck by the exaggeration of illness imposed by psychological factors. They often present our most challenging obstacles to achieving prescribed therapy. The potential role of emotional stress in cardiovascular disease has held my clinical and research interest for over a decade. Increasingly, my colleagues have encouraged me to express my views, conceptions and misconceptions regarding the current status of the role of emotional stress in coronary heart disease, sudden coronary death, and hypertension. Recently, there has been an extensive reassessment of complex clinical data, including risk factors, lifestyle, coronary "proneness" and rehabilitation. The true value of many of these factors is in question.

Certainly, the role of life-style in cardiovascular disease is new and ill-defined. At the moment, the application of selective prognostic indices to sociobiologic events remains an elusive challenge. All elements of the problem are not yet in place; nevertheless, there is a need to identify what is known, what can be done now, and what goals remain for the future. This book reviews several of the contemporary questions that face physicians and health professionals today. Among the questions addressed are these: What is the evidence that stress plays a role in coronary heart disease, sudden death, and hypertension? What is the status of the current risk factor dilemma in coronary heart disease? What new prognostic markers are available? And which methods are useful and practical in the diagnosis and management of stress in patients with major cardiovascular illnesses?

Awareness is basic to the development of insight, interventions, and ultimately, prevention. Although incompletely defined, the information in this text is directed toward clinical adjuncts that can promote the quality of life and the sense of well-being of those at risk of developing, or already experiencing, cardiovascular disorders. Often the psychosocial factors are the most crippling in our patients. If we succeed in improving the quality of life for some, we can more patiently await the verdict on the value of these manipulations toward improving the quantity of life.

At this writing, there are many signs that point toward the interest in, and the importance of, balancing the remarkable advances in technology and science with the humanistic art of medicine. Many new areas have developed that can enhance clinical effectiveness. The new dimension of behavioral medicine, for example, integrates many health care disciplines into a common framework. This approach offers a more balanced and comprehensive method for meeting the totality of human needs in both health and disease. If this book in any measure assists in achieving that balance, it will have accomplished its entire purpose.

RSE, 1979

ACKNOWLEDGEMENTS

Many friends and colleagues have provided support, enthusiasm, and motivation for this text. The author would like to recognize the Monsour Medical Foundation for providing a chair in Cardiovascular Medicine at the University of Nebraska Cardiovascular Center for the purpose of developing this text and other programs directed at developing a more comprehensive understanding of the role of lifestyle in cardiovascular disease. Key to the development of this grant were four physician brothers — the Monsours, Bill, Howard, Roy, and Bob. Support in obtaining the grant for this purpose was provided by Doctor Robert D. Sparks, former Chancellor of the University of Nebraska Medical Center, and currently Director of Health Programs for the W.K. Kellogg Foundation. Doctor Neal A. Vanselow, Chancellor of the University of Nebraska Medical Center, contributed to the momentum developed for this project by Doctor Sparks. I would also like to acknowledge the assistance of other members of the Monsour Medical Foundation — Doctor Robert Nossen, Miss Maureen Kroll, and Mr. Ben D. Razon — who reviewed manuscripts and provided significant support and direction for this project. The coordination of these activities was guided by the able hands of Rita Marchignoli.

Some of the dollars to underwrite the cost of this chair were provided for a medical editor, Ms. Emily Salhany. Unquestionably, her remarkable background in nutrition and medicine, as well as literature research, combined with her tireless optimism and careful attention to detail, has made the author's task an opportunity rather than a burden.

Many friends and colleagues supplied reprints and personal communications that are incorporated into this text. In addition, because of the variety of topics to be included, it was essential that each chapter receive outside review by one or more experts. With regard to review, the author would particularly like to acknowledge the assistance of Doctors Giorgio Baroldi, James C. Buell, Robert L. Grissom, Wesley E. Sime and Gerald Wolf. The chapter on "Behavioral Therapies" was greatly influenced by the input of Doctor Hermann Witte and Doctor Stephen Weiss. The chapter on "Family Life" was markedly influenced by Doctor Bruce Munro, whose international background and extensive clinical experience assisted in providing a succinct statement of the complex nature of family life today.

The preparation of the manuscript was a complex task involving a small army of secretaries, assistants, and even a teenage son. The troops included Vicki Aughe, Sheri Dunbar, Kay Exstrom, Holly Hughes, Becky Jacobs, Kris Jorgensen, Mona Montalvo, Jan Svec, Jim Ussery, Marie Wissig, and yes, William R. Eliot. The artwork and figures were developed by Roger Aughe, George Cave, Rose Reynolds, and Doctor Gordon Todd. The manuscript was proofread and reviewed by Alice Laski.

The author also recognizes the assistance of Mr. Steven Korn and Mr. Jacques Strauss of Futura Publishing Company, and Doctor Reba Benschoter of the Department of Biomedical Communications at the University of Nebraska Medical Center. The staff members of the Cardiovascular Center at the University of Nebraska Medical Center were very generous with their support, comments and willingness to provide services during occasional scheduled and unscheduled absences related to the preparation of this text. These include Doctor Alan Forker, Doctor James Buell, Doctor Barry Dzindzio, Doctor Robert Grissom, Doctor Helen Starke, and Mr. Ted Laski. Mr. James Ussery was of immeasurable assistance in a variety of ways in the writing and rewriting of the text.

Naturally, this kind of work does not get done without a great deal of support from the domestic unit. Leading in this category was my wife, Phyllis, who provided work space, moral support, meals, reviews, and a host of intangibles that created the appropriate chemistry for writing the book. In addition, my son, William, and my daughter, Susan, were remarkably understanding in that they made many concessions with regard to their friends, high fidelity systems, electric guitar and so forth to provide an atmosphere of quiet and contemplation. Finally, I would like to thank my friends Mr. Duane Acklie, Mr. John Delich, General Russell Dougherty, Mr. Don Leonard, Mr. Donald Lowe, Mrs. C. Louis Meyer, Mr. William Nelligan, Mrs. Mary Elaine O'Neal, Mr. Lou Somberg, and Mr. David Tews for their generous support. Special thanks are directed to the friends of Doctor Paul Burgert who gave memorial gifts that assisted in the cost of developing this text.

CHAPTER 1

ETIOLOGY

Everyone knows or thinks he knows what stress is. The perception of stress is highly individual. Frequently the differentiation between subjective and objective features of stress is a difficult if not impossible task. It is even more difficult to attempt to quantify the impact of an individual's stress response without considering the resilience or coping capabilities available. Thus, assigning numerical values to such sociobiologic events in stress-linked disease states is a goal yet to be achieved by clinical investigators.

Enough information from previous studies is available to attempt to define stress in contemporary terms for practical clinical purposes. An early and suitable, although restrictive, definition of stress was offered by Harold G. Wolff[1]: physical, psychological and symbolic stimuli capable of eliciting physiological responses. It can be argued that this definition of stress implies an inappropriate and perhaps destructive physiologic response, and that, to some extent, it does not take into consideration the fact that stress can be managed either in a supportive, reinforcing manner or in a self-destructive fashion. Hans Selye[2] further broadened the definition of stress by taking into consideration that stressful factors in the environment may or may not produce harmful effects. He considered the stimulus the stressor and the response the stress, and termed unproductive or self-destructive stress as distress, and productive or reinforcing stress as simply stress itself. He reinforced the concept that stress responses are part of the general adaptation syndrome, and it follows logically that life without stress is death. Selye[3] also placed emphasis on the inten-

1

sity of the demand for readjustment or adaptation, and felt
that it was unimportant whether the stressing agent, or
stressor, was pleasant or unpleasant. These concepts are
useful and practical in that they allow well recognized clinical differences in response to the same stress or stressor.

Earlier, Cannon[4] also had discussed the concept of
stress being the stimulus and strain the response. His major
contribution to the field was the concept of fight or flight,
wherein a stressful stimulus produces an alarm reaction in
the animal or individual as preparation for either fight or
flight.[5] Although an oversimplification, this concept has
considerable utility.

Recently, the First National Conference on Emotional
Stress and Heart Disease[6] has offered a more clinical definition: stress is "an obviously painful or adverse force which
induces distress or strain upon both the emotional and
physical makeup." The latter definition is a useful compila-
tion of previous and contemporary contributors.

It is my concept that stress is initiated by a highly complex mosaic of events which collectively recruit individual
coping abilities that are ultimately translated into constructive or destructive psychophysiologic responses. Fundamental to the contemporary understanding of stress is the
recognition of the rapid and remarkable change in the lifestyle of modern man and its potential influence on human
adjustment and behavior. The first is a dramatic increase in
the number of events, or stimuli, or stressors, to be
monitored by each individual on a daily or annual basis. It
has been suggested that contemporaries encounter one
thousand times the number of events per annum as were
experienced by their great grandparents. Some of these
events are produced by instantaneous communications systems such as the telephone, television and radio; the sense
of immediacy created by these systems imposes upon the
individual constant monitoring, evaluation and discrimina-
tion of the information received. Thus, a geographically
remote stimulus can set off a local alarm reaction. Today,

no one and no place is remote, unattackable, isolated, self-sufficient or "safe". The potential for travel in the twentieth century allows us to cover distances in one hour by jet which would have taken a month by wagon for the pioneers. Thus, within the last century, the number of events to be monitored has increased exponentially while the time for decision making has remained the same or has been shortened.

One of the major differences between us and our great grandparents is the relative absence of immediate threat to life. Even weather, shelter and hunger are lesser concerns in today's industrialized world. Yet, today we are often prohibited by society, bureaucracy, impaired communications or the sheer complexity of life from making prompt and appropriate decisions relative to perceived threats. Often the individual is held in a state of suspended animation, unable to physically resolve the inherent fight or flight dilemma. I refer to this unique twentieth century phenomenon as "invisible entrapment." In this situation, one may find oneself in a chronic alarm reaction, maintaining a constant state of visceral-vascular readiness for days, weeks, months or years. Thus, where life and death struggles were over within a matter of minutes previously, today's struggles may be suspended, unresolved and prolonged. Therefore, we can assume that the inborn alarm reaction for survival effective in the past has become, for some, a contemporary curse.

Cardiovascular conditions represent the major health problem of the industrialized world today. In the view of many investigators, life stress events which are a routine part of daily living can influence the susceptibility to illness.[7,8] Events such as the loss of a spouse, arguments with the boss, assumption of a large mortgage, and deadlines are among the risky events noted. Investigators frequently tie these life change events to the increased risk of cardiovascular disease in industrialized societies.[9-11] Such studies have been largely retrospective. Prospective investigations[12-14] have been less successful in predicting which individuals are at risk from increased life change events alone.

The layman's awareness of stress has been increased by the recent emphasis on this field. Awareness has always been an important preventive measure by offering the opportunity for individual preparation. Hopefully, the benefits of knowing both the constructive and destructive influences of stress can increase man's insight into preventable stress-linked conditions.

Some of the untoward effects of awareness include the avoidance of stress (the "drop out" response), which itself creates new forms of stress. Equally, there may be a preconditioned hyperalertness to stress, leading to overreaction. "Making mountains out of mole hills" usually precludes optimal solutions. For some individuals, denial is a useful defense mechanism.

As mentioned, the perception of events is a highly individual phenomenon — "one man's meat is another man's poison." It was indicated that Selye[3] defines stress as either positive and reinforcing or negative. It presents itself as either an opportunity or a problem and, thus, is influenced not only by the degree of stress present at any given time but also by the individual's perception and resilience.

A stressful event is not selective for any particular target organ. Target organ susceptibility is also based upon complex constitutional and/or acquired factors. Biochemical and physiologic responses are frequently unique and may not be uniform, even in the same individual. For example, anxiety tends to produce elevation of circulating epinephrine, whereas anger tends to elevate circulating norepinephrine levels.[15] Even cholesterol may be raised in response to chronic stress or acute stressful conditions. Corticosteroid changes are highly individual and inappropriate as screening tools or stress markers.[16] Twenty-four hour urine catecholamine assays have also been of dubious value.[17] Thus, a single chemical assay which labels the stress response remains an elusive target for clinical investigators.

In any environment there are always organisms or animals that are more capable of adapting to change. Undoubtedly there exist in twentieth century society "supermen" and "superwomen." These individuals probably have remarkable and appropriate coping mechanisms. Study of such individuals may reveal methods for developing optimal coping mechanisms that can be applied to the more susceptible or fragile members of our society. These methods might include strong support systems such as the family unit, mutually supportive work groups, or career flexibility. Development of these support systems requires the recruitment of individual, family and community resources to enhance the physician's role and effectiveness.

To understand how stress is handled, I have found it useful to employ the diagram shown in Figure 1-1. In viewing the response to a stimulus, there are three steps: first, the perception; second, the interpretive process; and third, response. Any event is perceived in the central nervous system by auditory, visual, tactile and/or enteroreceptors. The interpretation of what is perceived is based upon previous experience and a variety of individual factors which determine whether the stimulus represents a threat or not. The discriminating process will then reject nonthreatening situations and no response is required. When a threat is perceived, a response will be required which may not be optimal with regard to the individual's ego. As a result, it may or may not be personally acceptable as an option. When the response is one which is optimal to the individual, there can be a reinforcement or, as it is labeled by Selye,[3] "eustress." When it is suboptimal there may be strain. Each event can be considered individually, but the results are collective. As suboptimal responses accumulate, the individual's coping systems can become overloaded. An accumulation or acceleration of unresolved suboptimal responses induces a state of chronic visceral-vascular readiness. This phenomenon in animals predisposes to hypertension, myocardial infarction and peptic ulcer.

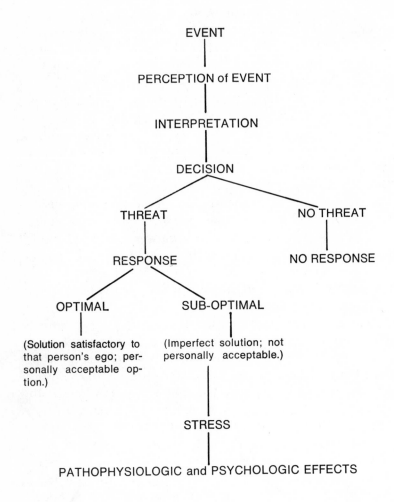

Figure 1-1. *Diagram depicting the manner in which stress is handled from the event itself, perception of the event, and interpretation leading to a decision. If the decision is made that the event is not a threat, no response is required. If the decision is that the event is a threat, the response may be either optimal (a personally acceptable option) or sub-optimal (not personally acceptable), which will be stressful and can lead to pathophysiologic and psychologic effects.*

In the physiologic sense, stress has been broadly defined by Gilmore[18] as "an adaptive response which prepares the organism for, or adapts it to, a given situation." He finds it convenient to view the response system from three aspects: first, the afferent or stimulus; second, the integrating process; and third, the efferent or response.[19] With respect to the former, the central nervous system receives a wide variety of inputs from auditory, visual and tactile receptors as well as from the enteroreceptors. From a practical standpoint, most of the integration of the stress reaction, or response, occurs in the hypothalamus and involves the coordination of all of the effector responses. These may be divided into the somatomotor, the hormonal and the visceral motor systems. There is an interplay between these three systems, in addition, which is based on feedback and complex interrelationships. Nevertheless, for the purposes of discussion they may be considered as three distinct units. There is evidence to suggest that both mental stress and exercise are mediated via the defense area in the hypothalamus.[20] Bulbring and Burn[21] have demonstrated that vasodilatation is blocked by atropine and is, therefore, mediated by sympathetic vasodilator nerves. Autoregulation of vasodilatation is controlled by hypothalamic stimulation.[22] Stimulation of the defense areas of the hypothalamus in the cat causes the alarm reaction with elevated aortic pressure, heart rate, contractile force and muscle blood flow, while renal blood flow diminishes.[23,24] Evidence suggests that chronic stimulation of this area in animals can lead to chronic hypertension.[25]

The work of Brod and associates[26] reveals the influence of emotional stress (arithmetic calculations timed with a metronome) on cardiac output, forearm blood flow and other hemodynamic parameters. During the arithmetic calculations (stimulus), muscle blood flow, cardiac output and renal resistance were shown to increase, whereas splanchnic blood flow decreased. Similar responses of cardiac output to mental stress have been reported by Hickam and associates[27] employing the ballistocardiogram. Thus, it is clear that cardiovascular changes integrated through the defense center of the hypothalamus induce a visceral vascular ready state in experimental animals, which in turn causes changes similar to those observed in human clinical studies.

Raab[28] and Selye,[29] among others, have identified the importance of the autonomic nervous system in the stress response. As a result of autonomic outflow, the adrenal medulla will be stimulated to produce epinephrine or norepinephrine or both. In addition, it has been suggested that chronic physical or emotional stress causes adrenal cortical overproduction of corticosteroids.[15] Steroid excess induces sodium and water retention, a well-recognized, pathophysiologic mechanism in several vascular conditions. Adrenal cortical stimulation is known to occur in response to a variety of psychosocial stimuli. The hypophyseal adrenal cortical system, however, reacts more slowly and requires somewhat higher stimulus intensities before reaction than does the hypothalamic adrenal medullary system.[30] Therefore, adrenal medullary excesses appear in acute stress syndromes, whereas adrenal cortical excesses would be expected in conditions of chronic stress. It has also been pointed out that a variety of psychosocial stimuli may elicit significant increases in thyroid function as measured by protein bound iodine.[30] Other indices of thyroxine release have been shown to be excessive in animals and in man under similar circumstances. It is unknown whether adrenal medullary cortical excess directly enhances adrenal cortical production and vice versa.

It is possible that the chronic stress reaction encompasses a series of homeostatic maladaptations. As mentioned earlier, the social impropriety of fight or flight precludes rapid resolution of the chronically overstimulated cardiovascular system. Instead, there is a socially enforced uncoupling between the heart and the musculoskeletal system. If this intense state of visceral-vascular readiness is sustained for prolonged periods of time, secondary systemic hypertension and tachyarrhythmias, for example, could result. Elevation of blood pressure has been observed in animals receiving electrical stimulation to the hypothalamus.[24] Hypertension has also been produced in animals by crowding.[31] It is thus proposed that in the chronic state of visceral vascular readiness there develops a progressive elevation or resetting of the baroreceptor system. These receptors then interpret normotension at progressively higher levels. In the initial phase, elevated blood pressure may be reduced by favorable manipulation of the external forces (environmental circumstances) underlying the chronic alarm reaction. Later, as the systems become more fixed, they require pharmacologic intervention.

Examples of environmentally induced hypertension may be found in the process of urbanization of the Zulu community.[32] Other examples of the role of environmental factors in hypertension include life threatening events such as the 1947 Texas City Crisis,[33] combat conditions in war[34] and others. The situation has been well summed up by Ostfeld and Shekelle[35]: "Contemporary man, in much of the world, is faced every day with people and with situations about which there is uncertainty of outcome, wherein appropriate behavior is not prescribed and validated by tradition, where the possibility of bodily or psychological harm exists, where running or fighting is inappropriate, and where mental vigilance is called for." These circumstances surround the contemporary epidemic of essential hypertension.

With chronic tachycardia, hypertension, increased cardiac output, elevated catecholamines, enhanced inotropy and other features of the alarm reaction, there are greatly increased demands for myocardial oxygenation. The chronic uncoupling of the cardiovascular system from the musculoskeletal system is the twentieth century "experiment" unique in human experience. The specific effects of chronic uncoupling of these systems are under investigation. The aforementioned conditions, however, are well recognized pathophysiologic components of a variety of cardiovascular catastrophes and disease states.

PSYCHOLOGICAL EFFECTS

In association with Warheit and others, we conducted an eight year study into the psychosocial aspects of cardiovascular disease affecting some of the employees at the Kennedy Space Center (KSC) in Florida. Our findings supported the view that there were abnormally high levels of coronary heart disease associated with untoward psychological distress among a sample of the ground support employees at the Space Center.[36] Empirical data from electrocardiographic tracings and mortality rates revealed that personnel at the Center were at unusually high risk with regard to coronary heart disease.[37] The data from psychiatric inventories combined with statistics on death rates by suicide demonstrated significantly higher levels of psychoneuroticism and suicide for the Kennedy Space Center (KSC) sample than for those of age and sex matched control groups from the general population (150 experimentals and 50 controls). However, when the data on specific occupations and psychoneuroticism was analyzed, significantly higher rates were found among KSC employees who were administrators, managers, and foremen, as compared to control samples.[38] This finding suggested that those in occupations involving management, coordination of tasks, or supervision of workers were experiencing circumstances which, in turn, may have become translated into unusually high levels of psychoneuroticism, particularly anxiety and depression. Of interest was the finding that the differences between the KSC and control groups were not significant for those with manual skills as compared with unskilled workers.

Data relating occupation, electrocardiographic abnormality and psychological distress to SMA 12 and complete blood count and blood pressures were not statistically significant.[37] Serum cholesterol levels and blood pressures were within normal limits for almost the entire KSC sample. These were singularly unrelated to electrocardiographic, psychoneurotic, or mortality data.[36]

Although the findings of this study were inconclusive, some of the evidence was very suggestive. This included occupational stress and its relationship to psychoneuroticism and coronary heart disease. However, no significant relationships were found between electrocardiographic features, high psychiatric symptom scores, blood chemistry aberrations or blood pressure variations.[36] The reasons for these disparate findings are not obvious. One can, however, offer some suggestions and observations regarding the question of occupational stress and its relationship to disease. Social, psychological and biological processes involved in any model of disease are extremely complex, even for those disorders having a clearly identifiable organic cause. When the primary etiologic agents include socioenvironmental and psychological factors, the web of interrelationships becomes highly complex and extremely difficult to untangle with available knowledge. A number of significant theoretical advances will be needed to determine these effects more accurately.

The data from KSC, however, suggests that socioenvironmental stressors were instrumental in either producing or provoking latent cardiovascular and psychoneurotic conditions among work groups.[36] The relationship between the various factors and the resultant processes leading from occupation to stress to disease and death could not be anticipated or clearly identified. In this sense, the research represents a microcosm of most of the stress research being conducted today, in that there are unmistakable clues which link socioenvironmental and social psychological stress to disease syndromes. Yet these factors are elusive.

As a physician and investigator, one could not overlook the high levels of anxiety, depresssion, alcoholism, divorce, and drug abuse in concert with a high incidence of sudden coronary death and acute myocardial infarction. Yet where was the pathophysiologic chain of responsible events? It was even more frustrating that these events did not correlate with the routine risk factors of hypercholesterolemia, hyperglycemia, hypertension, excessive cigarette usage and obesity.

It is painfully obvious that individual susceptibility is not measurable with static chemical or physiological parameters. Individualized emotional stress testing methods similar to exercise stress testing offer a hopeful approach which may have practical clinical impact.

REFERENCES

1. Wolff, H.G.: Life stress and bodily disease — A formulation. In H.G. Wolff, S.G., Wolf, Jr., and C.C. Hare (Eds.): *Life Stress and Bodily Disease*, Baltimore: Williams and Wilkins, Co., 1950, pp. 1059-1094.
2. Selye, H.: *The Stress of Life*, New York: McGraw-Hill, 1956.
3. Selye, H.: *Stress in Health and Disease*, Boston: Butterworth, Inc., 1976.
4. Cannon, W.B.: Stresses and strains of homeostasis. *Amer. J. Med. Sci.* **189**:1-14, 1935.
5. Cannon, W.B.: *Bodily Changes in Pain, Hunger, Fear and Rage*, New York: D. Appleton and Co., 1929.
6. Workshop IV: Emotional stress and coronary artery disease. *J. South Carolina Med. Assoc.* (Supplement) **72**:88-95, 1976.
7. Gunderson, E.K.E.: Introduction to E.K.E. Gunderson and R.H. Rahe (Eds): *Life Stress and Illness*, Springfield, Illinois: Charles C. Thomas, 1974, pp. 3-7.
8. Rahe, R.H., McKean, J.D., and Arthur, R.J.: A longitudinal study of life change and illness patterns. *J. Psychosomatic Res.* **10**:355-366, 1967.

9. Rahe, R.H., Romo, M., Bennett, L., and Siltanen, P.: Subjects' recent life changes, myocardial infarction and abrupt coronary death. *Arch. Intern. Med.* **133**:221-228, 1974.

10. Rahe, R.H., Arajarvi, H., Arajarvi, S., Punsar, S., and Karvonen, M.J.: Recent life changes and coronary heart disease in East versus West Finland. *J. Psychosomatic Res.* **20**:431-437, 1976.

11. Rahe, R.H.: Stress and strain in coronary heart disease. *J. South Carolina Med. Assoc.* (Supplement) **72**:7-14, 1976.

12. Goldberg, E.L., and Comstock, G.W.: Life events and subsequent illness. *Amer. J. Epidemiology* **104**:146-158, 1976.

13. Rahe, R.H.: The pathway between subjects' recent life changes and their near-future illness reports: Representative results and methodological issues. In B.S. Dohrenwend and B.P. Dohrenwend (Eds.): *Stressful Life Events,* New York: John Wiley and Sons, 1974, pp. 73-86.

14. Holmes, T.S.: *Adaptive Behavior and Health Change.* Medical thesis, University of Washington, Seattle, 1970.

15. Raab, W.: Emotional and sensory stress factors in myocardial pathology. *Amer. Heart J.* **72**:538-564, 1966.

16. Mason, J.W.: Emotion as reflected in patterns of endocrine integration. In L. Levi (Ed.): *Emotions — Their Parameters and Measurement,* New York: Raven Press, 1975, pp. 143-181.

17. Frankenhaeuser, M.: Experimental approaches to the study of catecholamines and emotion. In L. Levi (Ed.): *Emotions — Their Parameters and Measurement,* New York: Raven Press, 1975, pp. 209-234.

18. Gilmore, J.P.: Cardiovascular response to emotional stress. *J. South Carolina Med. Assoc.* (Supplement) **72**:27-32, 1976.

19. Gilmore, J.P.: Physiology of stress. In R.S. Eliot (Ed.): *Stress and the Heart,* Mt. Kisco, New York: Futura Publishing Co., 1974, pp. 69-90.

20. Eliasson, S., Lindgren, P., and Uvnas, B.: Representation in the hypothalamus and the motor cortex in the dog of the sympathetic vasodilator outflow to the skeletal muscle. *Acta Physiol. Scand.* **27**:18-37, 1952.

21. Bulbring, E., and Burn, J.H.: The sympathetic dilator fibres in the muscles of the cat and dog. *J. Physiol.* **83**:483-501, 1935.

22. Djojosugito, A.M., Folkow, B., Lisander, B., and Sparks, H.: Mechanism of escape of skeletal muscle resistance vessels from the influence of sympathetic cholinergic vasodilator fibre activity. *Acta Physiol. Scand.* **72**:148-156, 1968.

23. Rosen, A.: Augmented cardiac contraction, heart acceleration and skeletal muscle vasodilatation produced by hypothalamic stimulation in cats. *Acta Physiol. Scand.* **52**:291-308, 1961.

24. Feigl, E., Johannson, B., and Lofving, B.: Renal vasoconstriction and the defense reaction. *Acta Physiol. Scand.* **62**:429-435, 1964.

25. Herd, J.A., Morse, W.H., Kelleher, R.T., and Jones, L.G.: Arterial hypertension in the squirrel monkey during behavioral experiments. *Amer. J. Physiol.* **217**:24-29, 1969.

26. Brod, J., Fencl, V., Hejl, Z., and Jirka, J.: Circulatory changes underlying blood pressure elevation during acute emotional stress (mental and arithmetic) in normotensive and hypertensive subjects. *Clinical Science* **18**:269-279, 1959.

27. Hickam, J.B., Cargill, W.H., and Golden, A.: Cardiovascular reactions to emotional stimuli. Effect on the cardiac output, arteriovenous oxygen difference, arterial pressure, and peripheral resistance. *J. Clin. Invest.* **27**:290-298, 1948.

28. Raab, W.: *Preventive Myocardiology,* Springfield, Illinois: Charles C. Thomas, 1970.

29. Selye, H.: *The Physiology and Pathology of Exposure to Stress,* Montreal: Acta, Inc., 1950.

30. Levi, L.: Psychosocial stress and disease: A conceptual model. In E.K.E. Gunderson and R.H. Rahe (Eds.): *Life Stress and Illness,* Springfield, Illinois: Charles C. Thomas, 1974.

31. Henry, J.P., Meehan, J.P., and Stephens, P.M.: The use of psychosocial stimuli to induce prolonged systolic hypertension in mice. *Psychosomatic Med.* **29**:408-432, 1967.

32. Gampel, M.B., Slome, C., Scotch, N., and Abramson, J.H.: Urbanization and hypertension among Zulu adults. *J. Chronic Dis.* **15**:67-70, 1962.

33. Ruskin, A., Beard, O.W., and Schaffer, R.L.: "Blast hypertension." Elevated arterial pressures in the victims of the Texas City Disaster. *Amer. J. Med.* **4**:228-236, 1948.

34. Graham, J.D.P.: High blood pressure after battle. *Lancet* **248**:239-240, 1945.

35. Ostfeld, A.M., and Shekelle, R.B.: Psychological variables and blood pressure. In J. Stamler, R. Stamler, and T.N. Pullman (Eds.): *The Epidemiology of Hypertension,* New York: Grune and Stratton, 1967, pp. 321-331.

36. Warheit, G.J., and Eliot, R.S.: Unpublished work.

37. Reynolds, R.C.: Community and occupational influences in stress at Cape Kennedy. In R.S. Eliot (Ed.): *Stress and the Heart,* Mt. Kisco, New York: Futura Publishing Co., 1974, pp. 33-49.

38. Warheit, G.J.: Occupation: A key factor in stress at the Manned Space Center. In R.S. Eliot (Ed.): *Stress and the Heart,* Mt. Kisco, New York: Futura Publishing Co., 1974, pp. 51–65.

CHAPTER 2

RISK FACTORS

A review of observations, experiments and epidemiologic studies over the past 200 years has uncovered a wealth of knowledge but no solid evidence for the cause of coronary heart disease. A logical conclusion is that we have been seeking answers to the wrong questions in most cases. It is more likely, however, that the cause of coronary heart disease is highly complex and represents a mosaic, or perhaps even a continuum, of genetic and environmental factors which affect various degrees of vulnerability from one individual to the next. As has been recently pointed out, "Once the proper questions are asked and the relevant facts collected, any sensible person can reach the correct conclusions".[1] There are two limitations: the facts are never quite complete nor completely accurate;[3] and as Voltaire[2] pointed out, "Common sense is not so common."

Interest in the role of diet in heart disease was initiated by Gofman et al[4] in 1950, when they described a means for characterizing serum lipoproteins by ultracentrifugation. Later, Ancel Keys[5] concluded that the incidence of coronary heart disease in six countries was correlated with the available food fat. This was followed by two large prospective studies which attempted to determine the role of dietary habits in the etiology of coronary heart disease (Framingham and Tecumseh). In the Framingham study, a thousand persons were examined with a detailed dietary history. They were also examined for the incidence of hypertension, cigarette smoking, obesity, and sedentary lifestyle. Similar prospective studies were conducted in Tecumseh. In the Western Collaborative Group Study, the

aforementioned factors were reviewed in relation to behavior patterns (type A and type B of Rosenman and
Friedman) in a prospective sense.[6] Although the aforementioned list is not complete and the conclusions are highly
controversial, these studies, nevertheless, have dominated
current clinical recommendations and practices. For the
past decade, the public has received a large amount of information from the above sources, and many control and
prevention studies have been implemented. It has been im-
plied that control of these risk factors would lead to the
absence of coronary heart disease with the goal, it might be
concluded, that everyone would die of cancer.

Sensible management implies that the clinician under-
stands what is and what is not known in the field of risk,
prediction and coronary heart disease. It is, thus, of fundamental importance that current risk factors be placed in
practical perspective.

UTILITY OF RISK FACTORS

Before discussing the individual risk factors, let us step
back and attempt to view the entire gamut in an objective
and detached fashion. Several facts set the stage for future
discussion of individual factors. It has been well demonstrated that one cannot control an epidemic by merely treating the sick. It is obvious that a useful preventive program
must be applied. Prevention implies an understanding of
pathophysiology, which then leads to the logical question:
Do we understand the mechanisms? Clearly, the answer in
many cases is no. Subsequently, one must then query: Have
the right questions been asked? Disappointing answers to
this question can be found in studies where modification of
risk factors has been applied in populations with the hope
of reducing risk. For example, recent extensive studies in
Finland have failed to demonstrate a reversal of the coronary heart disease trend by strong application of risk factor

modification.[7] On my most recent visit to Finland as part of the Fourth Paavo Nurmi Symposium on sudden death, the clear indication of the Finnish investigators was that risk factor intervention at this point in time had not proven to be a successful venture.[8] In the United States, informal statements from key investigators revealed the frustration surrounding the Multiple Risk Factor Intervention Trial (MRFIT). Clearly what we have learned so far is how not to prevent coronary heart disease.

What is the problem? Are the risk factors inadequate? Are the intervention systems inappropriate? Are the investigators . . .?

Is there enough evidence, then, to warrant risk factor modification in clinical practice? In certain areas, the answer is a resounding yes. These areas, in order of priority, would include cigarette smoking, hypertension and weight control. The role of diabetes is less clear. No evidence has yet demonstrated the isolated contribution of a sedentary lifestyle. The most controversial factor at this time is the cholesterol hypothesis.

Although cause and effect relationships are unclear at this time, the predictive value, in a purely actuarial sense, of cigarette smoking, hypertension and obesity (when associated with another risk factor) is not only well known, but is an important rating practice of insurance companies. For example, control of cigarette smoking and hypertension has been followed by lowered incidence of disease and complications.[9-12] Still, the traditional risk factors are totally absent in more than half the new cases of coronary heart disease encountered in clinical practice.[13] Clearly, this demonstrates the need to seek new avenues toward the solution of the heart disease dilemma.

It is obvious, then, that there are other influences, risk factors, pathophysiologic mechanisms or whatever yet to be determined. Differences in cultures and societies are complicated, but the presence or absence of industrialization readily distinguishes the risk of coronary heart disease. The more industrialized the culture, the more it becomes at risk from coronary heart disease.[3] Therefore, risk factors must be considered in concert with the degree of industrialization of the society in question. The role of industrialized civilization needs to be better understood and more substantially clarified with regard to its impact on coronary heart disease.

MAJOR RISK FACTORS

Cholesterol

This factor was popularized in 1950 when Gofman et al[4] proposed that characterization of lipoproteins of blood serum by ultracentrifugation permitted two new contentions: (1) that low density lipoproteins were indicative of atherogenesis, and (2) that lipoprotein patterns could be favorably influenced by dietary manipulation. This diet heart hypothesis was followed by the globe trotting studies of Keys and associates.[5] In 1953, they concluded that fat in the diet correlated with coronary heart disease in six countries. The oversimplification of this hypothesis helped to rapidly develop it into a national dietary dogma. For many physicians, a low fat, low cholesterol diet prescription became as automatic in their treatment advice for heart disease as aspirin is for a headache.

The third phase of the cholesterol campaign ensued in 1967, when Fredrickson, Levy and Lees[14] promoted lipoprotein phenotyping of patients, employing Hatch's electrophoretic separation. Previous simple techniques were now complicated by new genetic terms, complexity and higher cost. Several investigations contradicted the report and determined it to be without genetic reality.[15,16] In my experience, phenotyping is rarely more helpful in management than standard blood cholesterol techniques. Albrink's[17] contention that hypertriglyceridemia is an independent contributor to atherogenesis and its complications has not been substantiated.[3] The latter was one of the fundamental tenets of the Fredrickson, Levy and Lees hypothesis.[14]

It is remarkably ironic that today there is a recent flurry of enthusiasm for a new contention diametrically opposed to the old, namely that high density lipoprotein levels are inversely proportional to the incidence of coronary heart disease.[18] This proposal had its origin in 1951 with the work of Barr, Russ and Eder,[19] which was ignored.

The Framingham study was conducted employing 1,000 persons who were examined with a detailed dietary interview. No evidence was found to support a relationship between dietary habits and cholesterolemia.[20] Two thousand persons were evaluated in the Tecumseh study in a similar fashion. Again, serum lipids were unrelated to dietary habits.[21] It is weakly argued that diets in the United States are so high in fat and cholesterol that they are above a so-called "critical threshold level", although the data does not seem to support this.[3]

It is frequently argued by the diet heart advocates that the reduction in coronary heart disease is the result of altered dietary habits. These statements disregard better coronary care units, better pre-hospital care of the potential coronary victim, increased interest in exercise conditioning, anti-smoking campaigns, and the control of hypertension by simple oral methods. Successful management of even a small percentage of the 60 million hypertensives in the United States could easily, by itself, influence these statistics. It has been pointed out that there is no evidence that cholesterolemia was diminished in the population of the United States during the interval from 1962 through 1973, the height of the diet heart disease campaign.[3]

Investigators have attempted to intervene utilizing both primary and secondary trials. In primary diet intervention, individuals are healthy and free of coronary disease; in the secondary trials, they are known to have coronary disease. With regard to these trials, Cornfield[22] has remarked that the better the trial design, the less well the diet treatment seems to work. An extensive Finnish trial on persons 34 to 64 years of age has revealed no effect of dietary intervention on total mortality — "Only an apparent influence on what the attending physicians thought the cause of death to be."[23,3]

It is also clear that animal experiments have little, if any, relevance to human experience. The production of atherosclerosis in animals by a variety of severe dietary alterations has brought little clarification to the understanding of human atherogenesis. It remains impossible to translate animal nutritional data into recommendations for human clinical practice.

It is possible to produce a more significant reduction in cholesterolemia by employing either niacin or clofibrate than by utilizing dietary intervention. Indeed, the cholesterol-lowering effects of these agents are about double those of the most rigorous dietary fat modifications.[24] No study has demonstrated a measurable effect on the incidence or the behavior of coronary heart disease by lowering serum cholesterol. Indeed, several drugs recommended for the control of cholesterol have led to excessive deaths or complications.[25-27] At present, there is no safe or efficacious agent available for the management of cholesterolemia.

Age influences the significance of hypercholesterolemia. In populations of men over 55, its predictive capability is insignificant.[3] In children with familial hypercholesterolemia, the risk of early coronary heart disease is greater, yet a suitable means for control remains to be found.[3] Here also, dietary intervention is of little assistance. A study of normal children has revealed no positive correlation between the level of serum cholesterol and dietary intake of calories, cholesterol, fat, saturated fat or sugar.[28]

We must still attempt to explain why serum cholesterol levels can be low in some individuals who die of typical myocardial infarction with extensive coronary atherosclerosis, why some can live beyond average life expectancy in the United States with high serum cholesterols, why cholesterol can become elevated more than a hundred milligrams percent in some certified public accountants from the first of January to the 15th of April, and why both emotional and physical stress can acutely elevate cholesterol.

It is a sobering thought that if a disease is common in a population, any other common environmental, chemical, or physiologic aberration will correlate to some degree with the occurrence of the disease. The risks for populations bear little relationship to the individual risk. Practical clinical techniques that are both sensitive and specific remain a challenge for future investigations. It is the clinicians and not the dogmatists who must practice with the inconclusive data supplied.

Hypertension

A host of actuarial tables support the validity of hypertension as a significant risk. At this point in the history of the United States, it is believed that approximately 35 million people have high blood pressure and that an additional 25 million may have intermittent, latent, hyperreactive or impending hypertension.[29] It is well accepted that the cause of hypertension can be found in less than 10 percent of all cases. The risk of hypertension in coronary heart disease is directly proportional to the mean arterial pressure and its duration. Arbitrary low risk limits for the diastolic levels have been said to be 90 to 100 mm Hg, and for systolic pressure it has been commonly understood that 100 mm Hg plus the individual's age is a low risk limit. Considerable modification of these criteria has been accomplished over the past four to five years. It is now believed, for example, that elderly individuals with elevated systolic blood pressure may be at increased risk owing to the sustained high mean arterial pressure. Thus, this form of hypertension is deserving of more clinical attention and therapy. In younger individuals, sustained elevations of blood pressure can be shown to accelerate the atherosclerotic process, perhaps by the introduction of mechanical trauma to the intimal surface of large and small arteries. Small vessel changes increase peripheral resistance, thereby enhancing left ventricular afterload. Subsequently, left ventricular hypertrophy, cardiac failure, and renal complications can be expected.

Although hypertension has been shown to be a significant risk factor, its control is of debatable value in reducing the incidence of coronary heart disease, namely myocardial infarction or sudden death. Antihypertensive therapy, however, significantly reduces the risk of cerebrovascular accidents, dissecting aneurysm, congestive failure and renal disease.[11,12] The failure to reduce the incidence of acute myocardial infarction and sudden coronary death has been a therapeutic enigma until recently.

It has been suggested that static determinations of blood pressure are of less importance to sudden death and acute myocardial infarction than dynamic changes within normal or abnormal ranges. That is, a sudden increase in blood pressure in a hypertensive individual can occur in the presence of therapeutic agents designed to produce a static reduction in blood pressure.[30] These would include diuretics, primarily. New Swedish work supports the aforementioned hypothesis, in that utilization of propranolol in the management of hypertension has been shown to reduce the incidence of coronary heart disease.[31]

Cigarette Smoking

Cigarette smoking markedly increases the risk of coronary heart disease and the degree of cigarette smoking is directly proportional to the risk.[9] Cigarette smoking is the clearest marker for coronary heart disease, although the mechanism is not understood. It is known that carbon monoxide can reduce myocardial oxygenation owing to the affinity of hemoglobin for carbon monoxide (about 240 times greater than the affinity of hemoglobin for oxygen). Carbon monoxide also may be incorporated into cardiac myoglobin, thereby decreasing the potential for oxygen transport from blood to the myocardium. Animals raised in a carbon monoxide atmosphere display a higher incidence of atherosclerosis.[32] Nicotine, also, is a component of tobacco, and among its actions are the release of catecholamines and the stimulation of the sympathetic system.

It is well to question the role of individual behavioral factors that can influence the need to smoke. "Surely, one must always consider the crucial question of whether the smoker or the smoking is the culprit."[33] Do those who smoke for some genetic, constitutional, or behavioral reason display an increase in coronary heart disease? Do they smoke to fill a need unique to their behavioral configuration? Do they have a higher level of emotional stress and tension than those who can either resist smoking initially or discontinue it? Recent German investigations reveal that heavy cigarette smokers are much younger at the time of acute myocardial infarction.[34] It is yet to be determined whether the cessation of cigarette smoking reduces coronary heart events as a result of chemical or behavioral adjustments. Serial coronary angiographic studies have clearly revealed the role of smoking in the acceleration of coronary atherosclerosis over all other risk variables.[35] Thus, from a practical clinical standpoint, discontinuance of cigarette smoking remains the most powerful preventive tool, whatever the physiologic mechanism.

Diabetes Mellitus

In the search for causes of heart disease, it is difficult to consider diabetes mellitus a risk factor in itself. For the person with diabetes, coronary heart disease is certainly more frequent; but for the population at large, diabetes cannot be considered a risk in itself. The reasons for the higher incidence of atherosclerosis associated with diabetes await the understanding of the pathophysiology of diabetes itself. The ability to reduce atherosclerosis by better control of the condition remains an important research goal. Unfortunately, optimal control is not associated with the reversal, or even the cessation, of the atherogenic process. Diabetes appears to accelerate the atherosclerotic process, thereby contributing to the "'premature" emergence of coronary heart disease.

Family History

Family history of coronary heart disease has been associated with an increased coronary risk. The basis is hypothesized to be genetic predisposition by itself or related to one of the other genetic risk factors such as hypertension or hypercholesterolemia. It is difficult to separate nature and nurture. Lifestyle, similar strivings, similar diet in similar environmental circumstances, all may lead to similar habits and similar risks on an environmental basis, rather than on a genetic basis. Frequently, the occurrence of coronary heart disease in offspring may even antedate the development in parents. It can be said that a family history is important, but it must be balanced with environmental circumstances.

Obesity

It frequently comes as a surprise to clinicians that exogenous obesity, without associated risk factors, is not a proven and significant risk factor in coronary heart disease.[36–40] Yet actuarial tables demonstrate the association between obesity and premature death from a number of causes. It will be recalled that reduction in body weight is often a successful treatment adjunct in the control of hyper-

lipidemia and hypertension.[41] In reality, obesity contributes to, and increases the risk of, coronary heart disease
whenever it is associated with any other accepted risk factor
such as cigarette smoking or hypertension.

Undefined Potential Risks

Currently, medical research is focusing attention upon
other factors which are believed to play significant roles in
coronary heart disease. These risk factors are most commonly observed in industrialized societies where coronary
heart disease is rampant. They include emotional stress,
behavior patterns, anxiety, depression, neuroticism and life
changes. It is an optimistic note that the current controversy
over the risk factors is leading to the development of new
research teams asking fresh research questions — a healthy
sign for the future of science.

REFERENCES

1. Greenwood, M., cited by Mann, G.V.-Diet-heart: End of an
   era. *New Eng. J. Med.* **297**:644-650, 1977.
2. Voltaire, F.M.A.: *Dictionnaire Philosophique,* 1764.
3. Mann, G.V.: Diet-heart: End of an era. *New Eng. J. Med.*
   297:644-650, 1977.
4. Gofman, J.W., Lindgren, F., Elliott, H., et al: The role of
   lipids and lipoproteins in atherosclerosis. *Science* **111**:166-
   171, 1950.
5. Keys, A.: Atherosclerosis: A problem in newer public health.
   J. M. Sinai Hosp. **20**:118-139, 1953.
6. Rosenman, R.H., Brand, R.J., Jenkins, C.D., et al: Coronary
   heart disease in the Western Collaborative Group Study.
   Final follow-up experience of 8½ years. *J.A.M.A.* **233**:872-
   877, 1975.
7. Puska, P., Tuomilehto, J., and Salonen, J.: Community control of acute myocardial infarction in Finland. *Practical Cardiology* **4**:94-100, 1978.

8. Romo, M.: Personal communication. September, 1977.
9. Kahn, H.A.: The Dorn study of smoking and mortality among U.S. veterans. *National Cancer Institute Monographs* **19**:1-125, 1966.
10. Hammond, E.C.: Smoking in relation to the death rates of one million men and women. *National Cancer Institute Monographs* **19**:127-204, 1966.
11. Veterans Administration Cooperative Study Group on Antihypertensive Agents: Effects of treatment on morbidity in hypertension. I. Results in patients with diastolic blood pressures averaging 115-129 mm Hg. *J.A.M.A.* **202**:1028-1034, 1967.
12. Veterans Administration Cooperative Study Group on Antihypertensive Agents: Effects of treatment on morbidity in hypertension. II. Results in patients with diastolic blood pressure averaging 90-114 mm Hg. *J.A.M.A.* **213**:1143-1152, 1970.
13. Keys, A., Aravanis, C., Blackburn, H., et al: Probability of middle-aged men developing coronary heart disease in five years. *Circulation* **45**:815-828, 1972.
14. Fredrickson, D.S., Levy, R.I., and Lees, R.S.: Fat transport in lipoproteins — An integrated approach to mechanisms and disorders. *New Eng. J. Med.* **276**:34-44, 94-103, 148-156, 215-225, 273-281, 1967.
15. Wada, M., Komoda, M., Mise, J.I., et al: Repeatability of the electrophoretic profiles of serum lipoproteins in hyperlipidemic subjects. *Japanese J. Clin. Pathol.* **24**:581-584, 1976.
16. Murphy, E. A.: *The Logic of Medicine,* Baltimore: Johns Hopkins University Press, 1976.
17. Albrink, M.J.: Triglycerides, lipoproteins, and coronary artery disease. *Arch. Intern. Med.* **109**:345-359, 1962.
18. Gordon, T., Castelli, W.P., Hjortland, M.C., et al: High density lipoprotein as a protective factor against coronary heart disease. The Framingham study. *Amer. J. Med.* **62**:707-714, 1977.
19. Barr, D.P., Russ, E.M., and Eder, H.A.: Protein-lipid relationships in human plasma. II. In atherosclerosis and related conditions. *Amer. J. Med.* **11**:480-493, 1951.

20. Kannel, W.B., and Gordon, T.: *The Framingham Diet Study: Diet and the Regulation of Serum Cholesterol (Section 24)*, Washington D.C.: Department of Health, Education and Welfare, 1970.

21. Nichols, A.B., Ravenscroft, C., Lamphiear, D.E., et al: Daily nutritional intake and serum lipid levels: The Tecumseh Study. *Amer. J. Clin. Nutrition* **29**:1384-1392, 1976.

22. Cornfield, J., and Mitchell, S.: Selected risk factors in coronary disease: Possible intervention effects. *Arch. Environmental Health* **19**:382-394, 1969.

23. Miettinen, M., Turpeinen, O., Karvonen, M.J., et al: Effect of cholesterol-lowering diet on mortality from coronary heart disease and other causes: A twelve year clinical trial in men and women. *Lancet* **2**:835-838, 1972.

24. National Diet-Heart Study Research Group: Final report. *Circulation* **37** :Supplement 1:1-419, 1968.

25. Coronary Drug Project Research Group. The Coronary Drug Project: Initial findings leading to modifications of its research protocol. *J.A.M.A.* **214**:1303-1313, 1970.

26. Coronary Drug Project Research Group: The Coronary Drug Project: Findings leading to further modifications of its protocol with respect to dextrothyroxine. *J.A.M.A.* **220**:996-1008, 1972.

27. Coronary Drug Project Research Group: The Coronary Drug Project: Findings leading to discontinuation of the 2.5 mg/day estrogen group. *J.A.M.A.* **226**:652-657, 1973.

28. Weidman, W.H., Elveback, L.R., Nelson, R.A., et al: Nutrient intake and serum cholesterol level in normal children 6 to 16 years of age. *Pediatrics* **61**:354-359, 1978.

29. Ward, G.W.: Info memo. National High Blood Pressure Education Program. National Heart, Lung, and Blood Institute. Department of Health, Education, and Welfare. Number 13, May 1978.

30. Bock, K.D., and Kreuzenbeck, W.: Spontaneous blood pressure variations in hypertension; The effect of therapy and correlation with complications. In F. Gross (Ed.): *Antihypertensive Therapy, Principles and Practice*, Berlin: Springer-Verlag, 1966, pp. 224-237.

31. Berglund, G., Sannerstedt, R., and Andersson, O.: Coronary heart-disease after treatment of hypertension. *Lancet* **1**:1-5, 1978.

32. Astrup, P.: Carbon monoxide and peripheral arterial disease. *Scand. J. Clin. Lab. Invest.* **19**: Supplement 99: 193-197, 1967.

33. Borhani, N.O.: Primary prevention of coronary heart disease: A critique. *Amer. J. Cardiol.* **40**:251-259, 1977.

34. Schettler, G., and Nussel, E.: Risk factors of coronary heart disease: New results in the Federal Republic of Germany. *Giron. Ital. Card.* **4**:366-372, 1974.

35. Gaarder, T.D., and Schwartz, D.C.: Influence of cigarette smoking on the natural history of coronary artery disease. *American College of Cardiology Extended Learning (ACCEL tape)* 10, Number 5, May, 1978.

36. Heyden, S., Hames, C.G., Bartel, A., et al: Weight and weight history in relation to cerebrovascular and ischemic heart disease. *Arch. Intern. Med.* **128**:956-960, 1971.

37. Kannel, W.B., Le Bauer, E.J., Dawber, T.R., et al: Relation of body weight to development of coronary heart disease. *Circulation* **35**:734-744, 1967.

38. Paffenbarger, R.S., Jr., Wolf, P.A., Notkin, J., et al: Chronic disease in former college students. I. Early precursors of fatal coronary heart disease. *Amer. J. Epidemiol.* **83**:314-328, 1966.

39. Chapman, J.M., Coulson, A.H., Clark, V.A., et al: The differential effect of serum cholesterol, blood pressure and weight on the incidence of myocardial infarction and angina pectoris. *J. Chronic Dis.* **23**:631-645, 1971.

40. Rosenman, R.H., Friedman, M., Straus, R., et al: Coronary heart disease in the Western Collaborative Group Study: A follow-up experience of 4 and one-half years. *J. Chronic Dis.* **23**:173-190, 1970.

41. Mann, G.V.: The influence of obesity on health. *New Eng. J. Med.* **291**:178-185, 226-232, 1974.

CHAPTER 3

PATHOPHYSIOLOGIC MECHANISMS

Acute myocardial infarction, sudden coronary death and hypertension are the major factors in cardiovascular death and disability. It is becoming apparent that mechanisms of acute myocardial infarction and sudden "coronary" death appear to be quite distinct. In hypertension, an organic cause is detected in less than 10 percent of the cases. In view of the newly recognized pathophysiologic impact of environmental and subjective influences, it is important to clarify the current pathophysiologic concepts.

PATHOPHYSIOLOGY OF CORONARY HEART DISEASE

As mentioned, it is likely that sudden coronary death and acute myocardial infarction are usually separate and distinct. The mechanism of acute myocardial infarction is incompletely defined and remains controversial. The inconsistent relationship between complete coronary arterial obstruction and acute myocardial infarction challenges the concept that arterial obstruction is a fundamental prerequisite to infarction. In 1912, Herrick[1] presented his classic paper on the clinical and pathologic features of myocardial infarction. Although emphasizing the role of coronary thrombosis, he clearly indicated that myocardial infarction did not always occur in animals or individuals experiencing sudden or chronic coronary arterial obstruction. In his time, however, the coronary circulation was believed to be an end-arterial system. This led to the conclusion that arterial blockage was the sine qua non of both sudden coronary death and myocardial infarction. On that basis, a variety of pathogenic mechanisms causing obstruction at any level of the coronary tree were proposed. The most frequent hypothetical mechanism was, and remains today, acute coronary thrombosis of the epicardial coronary vessels. Several investigators, however, have questioned the primary role of coronary thrombosis.[2-5] It is proposed that in many instances coronary thrombosis may, indeed, be a secondary event. Even secondary thrombus formation itself has been re-challenged. Thus, the stage is set for the current pathophysiologic controversy.

Coronary Thrombosis

The evidence suggests that if an individual experiences the typical onset of crushing substernal pain and dies early, coronary thrombosis will be a rare and unusual event.[6] On the other hand, should the same individual live to 72 hours, the presence of coronary thrombosis is a more likely event.[7] In the study of pathologic material from 100 consecutive autopsies on individuals who died within 25 days of the onset of such symptoms, 93 percent demonstrated old severe stenosis or complete obstruction of one or more of the major epicardial coronary vessels.[5] An acute thrombus was found in only 38 percent. The temporal relationships, as mentioned above, revealed that the longer the duration of symptoms before death, the more likely would be the presence of a thrombus. Similar studies have supported this position.

The key points revealed by this type of investigation are that: (1) in approximately seven percent of the individuals with typical acute myocardial infarction, no coronary occlusion is observed and minimal or no coronary luminal narrowing is present;[5] (2) in more than 60 percent of the infarctions there is no acute coronary thrombosis;[5] (3) all thrombi were found in vessels with atherosclerotic lumen reduction of at least 70 percent;[5] (4) the longer the stenotic segment, the more likely it was to be associated with coronary thrombosis;[5] (5) the larger the size of the myocardial infarction, the more likely a thrombus would be found in the associated epicardial coronary vessel;[5] (6) the amount of atheromatous material in the damaged vessel appeared to be directly proportional to the likelihood of a thrombus;[5] (7) there was a strong correlation between severe coronary stenosis and the enlargement of existing collateral vessels;[8] (8) the more severe the stenosis, the greater the development of collateral circulation serving the nearly or completely obstructed area;[8] (9) the same development of collateral circulation could be seen in coroners' cases of those who died of causes unrelated to cardiovascular disease and without previous history of coronary heart disease;[8] and (10) an occlusive coronary thrombus is never found in a normal coronary artery.[5] In summary, such findings indicate that an acute myocardial infarction occurs most often in individuals who experience pain for more than 24 hours before death and who have an old severe coronary obstruction and enlarged collateral vessels.

Studies utilizing radioisotopic fibrinogen injected into patients during the acute phase of myocardial infarction have also supported the possibility that coronary thrombosis is frequently a secondary event in certain instances.[9,10] In those who died of myocardial infarctions and displayed coronary thrombus, radioisotopic activity was incorporated into the thrombotic occlusion. The latter, of course, suggests that the coronary thrombus often develops subsequent to the initiation of the acute myocardial infarction. Also, in the view of several cardiac pathologists, the histology of the acute coronary thrombus postdates the pathologic landmarks of acute myocardial necrosis.[2,4,5] Remembering that coronary thrombus is absent in approximately 60 percent of all infarctions, its occurrence on a secondary basis must be considered among other possibilities. Finally, the presence of typical myocardial infarction, in the total absence of coronary disease or in the presence of minimal luminal narrowing, further excludes the thrombus from universal responsibilities for acute myocardial infarction.

Hemorrhage into an Atheromatous Plaque

In the early twentieth century, Paterson[11] described hemorrhage into an atheromatous plaque as a proposed mechanism and precursor for acute coronary arterial obstruction and subsequent myocardial infarction. It is found in a variety of pathologic settings. First, it is relatively frequently observed in coroners' cases in deaths unrelated to a cardiovascular cause.[12] In addition, it is a frequent finding (up to 22 percent) in syndromes of acute myocardial infarction.[12] Hemorrhage into an atheromatous plaque is occasionally found in association with an acute thrombosis.[12]

If the hemorrhage into an atheromatous plaque was to be considered a significant antecedent to acute myocardial infarction, there would be an extrusion of the atheromatous plaque and a resultant dislodging of atheromatous and cholesterol materials into the coronary lumen. Certain histopathologic features would be expected. First, one should find cholesterol or atheromatous emboli in distal portions of the coronary tree. There is little evidence that this occurs. Second, Herculean hemodynamic forces would be required for extrusion of an atheromatous plaque by the delicate vasa vasora. These atheromatous plaques are of considerable mass and attach themselves with great tenacity to the walls of the epicardial vessels. Hemodynamically-induced disruption would represent a true David and Goliath phenomenon. Some investigators believe that the process of hemorrhage into an atheromatous plaque followed by "healing" is part of the ever-changing atherogenic process. Nevertheless, it is a frequent finding in autopsies conducted in deaths from heart disease or unrelated causes. Thus, it remains an interloper in morbid coronary anatomy of nebulous pathophysiologic significance.

Presence of Old Obstruction

Evidence suggests that coronary atherosclerosis is a process which begins very early in life, as demonstrated by lipid streaks in the intimal portion of the fetus. The studies on relatively young U.S. soldiers killed in action in Korea supported this concept with an incidence of coronary atherosclerosis approximating 77 percent.[13] In an extensive study of individuals who died of unrelated cardiovascular causes, the incidence of coronary obstruction of one or more vessels approximated 37 percent.[14] Thus, there is evidence that coronary obstruction need not preclude a normal life span. Indeed, the aforementioned study implies that nearly two-fifths of the "healthy" population have silent coronary obstruction. This suggests that there is a normal life expectancy in a large percentage of the population in the presence of severe coronary obstruction. It can, therefore, be concluded that obstruction may or may not be associated with normal life expectancy and/or coronary heart disease. Obviously, elusive noncoronary arterial factors are playing important roles.

Small Vessel Disease

If one remains convinced that obstruction is the universal precursor to infarction, the last bastion of defense for this conviction is the myocardial microcirculation — small vessels. In recent years, it has been proposed that platelet aggregates can block the circulation in small vessels or at capillary levels. Platelet aggregate formation is encouraged at atherosclerotic luminal surfaces of the epicardial coronary vessel. It has thus been suggested that embolization of these aggregates would induce myocardial necrosis. In documented reports, however, only examples of isolated small vessel obstruction can be found. These are associated with conduction disturbances and cardiac arrhythmias.[15] There is no evidence for the development of typical coagulation necrosis, the hallmark of acute myocardial infarction. Yet another experiment of nature argues against the exclusive small vessel hypothesis. The disease thrombotic thrombocytopenic purpura is associated with profound hemolysis leading to hypoxia. Hemoglobin levels are frequently reduced to 25 percent of normal. In the terminal phase there is widespread aggregation and embolization of the myocardial small vessels. Despite these profound changes, microfocal coagulation necrosis is a rare occurrence in the terminal picture.[16]

When associated with acute myocardial infarction, small vessel disease is of a distinctly different secondary pathophysiologic variety. Following infarction, the adjacent small vessels are secondarily blocked with platelet thrombi. These findings are simultaneous with the revascularization phase of infarction, and are thus late and more apt to be secondary to impeded flow into the infarcted area.[8] Small vessel disease has also been reported employing myocardial biopsy. There is reported to be hyperplasia of the media with longitudinal disposition of the smooth muscle and progressive fibrosis of both media and intima. These are frequent findings in the trabeculae carneae and papillary muscles and are less often described in the interventricular septum. Almost all such reports are the result of right ventricular biopsies. Postmortem studies, however, indicate that identical histopathologic features are frequently displayed by healthy victims of non-cardiac deaths.[8] Furthermore, isolated right ventricular myocardial infarction is a practically nonexistent human event. The evidence is thus trivial for the role of small vessel disease in typical myocardial infarction or sudden death.

Normal Coronary Vessels

Postmortem pathologic proof of the incidence of normal coronary vessels and acute myocardial infarction has been offered by several investigators.[8,17-19] In a study of

100 autopsies from consecutive coronary care unit deaths from acute myocardial infarction, the incidence of normal vessels with minimal or no luminal narrowing was seven percent.[5] The clinical syndrome of ischemic heart disease with normal coronary vessels has been recognized since the early 1960s and has been supported by observations in both clinical and pathologic settings. The argument that a thrombus is formed in life but dissolved before death is unsupported by residual morphologic intimal damage from antecedent thrombi. Such features would not have been missed by the technique of Eliot and Baroldi.[17] Hypotheses to account for these unusual cases are numerous, yet none is universally acceptable at this writing.

The Role of Spasm

In the presence of minimal or no coronary luminal obstruction, it is logical that spasm would be offered as a pathophysiologic explanation for infarction. Interest has been enhanced as a result of the imaging by angiography of coronary spasm in cases of typical or Prinzmetal's angina.[20] However, it remains to be shown that spasm precedes or follows typical anginal pain and, if it does, what is the incidence and frequency of these events? In the meantime, it is difficult to accept spasm as the single cause of sudden coronary death or myocardial infarction in these instances because of a number of factors. First, the best physiologic coronary vasodilator is hypoxia. Second, animal studies indicate that coronary occlusion must be conducted for at least 60 minutes to experimentally produce a finite infarction.[21] Third, to conclude that spasm is a valid mechanism, it is necessary to record the chronologic events of spasm followed by electrophysiologic or hemodynamic derangement, followed then by the relief of spasm and, secondarily, the relief of the electrophysiologic and/or hemodynamic changes. The angiographic demonstration of coronary spasm subsequent to hemodynamic or electrophysiologic alterations is inadequate to prove cause and effect for the aforementioned reasons.[22] Equally, the disappearing thrombus theory or platelet aggregate embolization in normal vessels remains to be proven.

In the extensive experience of Gensini[23] and others, coronary spasm has been found to be an interloper in coronary angiography.[24,25] Most often it bears no detectable subjective or objective significance. Thus, the role of spasm remains to be proven.

Other Theories

Many other theories have been offered to explain myocardial ischemia and infarction; these include the myocardial "steal" syndrome, coronary hypotension, cardiac hypertrophy and deranged oxygen transport. The latter has been shown to induce myocardial necrosis in animals with normal coronary vasculature.[26,27] In the clinical setting, each hypothesis requires a more substantial background of supporting data. It seems most likely that a multifactorial mosaic of factors and events selectively operates in different individuals at different times to produce infarction.

Contrary to earlier opinion, the heart is not an end-arterial system lending itself readily to infarction by simple occlusion. Instead, a rich system of collateral vessels pervades the myocardium. Thus, as reviewed earlier, gradual occlusion of an extramural vessel is not necessarily followed by infarction. In many instances, it is believed that the collateral circulation prevents such an occurrence. Indeed, the development of coronary stenosis is paralleled by the opening of indigenous collateral circulation. The stimulus for collateral development has been shown by Barmeyer[28] to relate to stenosis or chronic hypoxia. In the former, the pressure gradient across the stenosis is the critical factor; in the latter, sustained chronic hypoxia (not intermittent), which can occur in such conditions as life at high altitude or anemia, is the critical factor. Because exercise conditioning is not a 24-hour daily phenomenon, it does not fulfill either of the aforementioned criteria for collateral formation.

In myocardial necrosis, the inner third of the left ventricle (referred to in this text as the subendocardium) is almost always involved. The two major types of myocardial infarction are transmural and nontransmural, and either can range from massive to minimal. Nontransmural infarctions tend to cluster in the midcardiac and subendocardial regions. The nearly inevitable involvement of the subendocardial region in acute myocardial infarction implies that it contains unique factors predisposing to myocardial necrosis.

Certain features render the subendocardial region the most frequent myocardial region to undergo ischemic necrosis. For example, by direct measurement, it has the lowest tissue partial pressure of oxygen of any organ or any layer of the heart. In this region, mechanical stress is the highest and myofibril lengths the longest, making oxygen demand the greatest. Other reported contributory factors include a capillary bed performing at near capacity at rest and myocardial blood flow dependent on diastole. Obviously, any tachycardia can limit the time available for coronary perfusion. Increased afterload from any cause, including chronic hypertension, will increase myocardial oxygen demands (MVO_2) and gradually increase myocardial tissue mass imposing further distribution difficulties. Oxygen transport factors such as anemia, carboxyhemoglobin, and hemoglobinopathies also predispose to myocardial ischemia or necrosis. Even endogenous catecholamines participating in the alarm reaction markedly increase MVO_2 by a variety of the aforementioned mechanisms.

Thus, there is evidence for a unique predisposition of the subendocardium to necrosis. When compared to the right ventricle, an interesting "control" experiment of nature can be found. The right ventricle almost never undergoes any form of isolated myocardial infarction (transmural or nontransmural). In order to produce isolated right ventricular myocardial infarction in animals, it is necessary, first, to induce pulmonary hypertension followed by marked right ventricular hypertrophy and, second, to ligate the right coronary epicardial vessel. These laboratory experiments do not find frequent clinical counterparts. It is, of course, well known that the right ventricle may be involved in myocardial infarction by extension from the left ventricle. In my experience, I have never seen an isolated transmural or nontransmural infarction of the right ventricle. Obviously, its pressure work requirements, coronary architecture, muscle mass, and a variety of other factors are more resistant to ischemic necrosis. Therefore, if Saint Peter gives you a choice of infarction, you might select an isolated transmural right ventricular variety.

Proposed Mechanism for Acute Myocardial Infarction

In view of the aforementioned observations, it is reasonable to consider alternatives to earlier concepts of the pathophysiology of acute myocardial infarction. It should be understood that much experimentation and controversy must be resolved before the appropriate answer will be known.

As reviewed, the inner third of the left ventricle (subendocardium) is uniquely vulnerable to myocardial necrosis. It is also known that there are a variety of factors that predispose it to myocardial infarction. As has been indicated, acute coronary obstruction does not appear to precede myocardial infarction in a significant number of patients. Therefore, it may be reasonable to assume that acute myocardial infarction is initiated through a myocardial mechanism which can be intensified under certain conditions by secondary coronary obstruction.

In making this assumption, let us consider a mosaic of chronic and acute pathophysiologic factors focusing at a

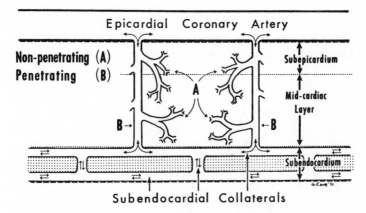

Figure 3-1. *Schematic showing the normal myocardial circulation. (A) Nonpenetrating coronary arteries. (B) Penetrating coronary arteries. Arrows demonstrate real and potential coronary flow. Reprinted with permission from Eliot, R.S., and Holsinger, J.W.: The pathophysiologic panorama of myocardial ischemia and infarction. In J.H.K. Vogel (Ed.):* Myocardial Infarction: A New Look at an Old Subject, *Advances in Cardiology, Volume 9, Basel: S. Karger AG, 1973, pp. 2-15.*

given point in time on the myocardium. Emotional shock, for example, is often accompanied by tachycardia, acutely elevated peripheral resistance, and catecholamine release as part of the contemporary alarm reaction. Factors of increased inotropism, decreased diastolic filling time, carboxyhemoglobin, increased wall tension, etc., may be focused upon the most vulnerable part of the left ventricle, the subendocardium. It is well known, from human and animal studies, that the loss of myocardial contractility in the first phase of myocardial ischemia may lead to myocardial necrosis unless one or more of the offending factors is eliminated within a reasonable period of time. Earlier, it was pointed out that coronary circulation is composed of external epicardial vessels, nonpenetrating and penetrating vessels interconnected with an extensive microcirculatory system (Figure 3-1). In the early phase of myocardial

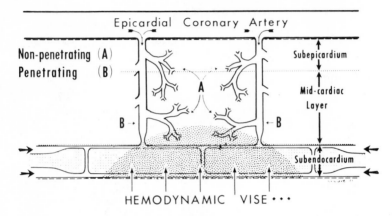

Figure 3-2. *Schematic depicting subendocardial ischemia. The stippled area represents subendocardial ischemia leading to oblitera-tion of the microcirculation. (A) Nonpenetrating coronary arteries. (B) Penetrating coronary arteries. Arrows demonstrate real and potential coronary flow. Reprinted with permission from Eliot, R.S. and Holsinger, J.W.: The pathophysiologic panorama of myocar-dial ischemia and infarction. In J.H.K. Vogel (Ed.):* Myocardial Infarction: A New Look at an Old Subject, *Advances in Car-diology, Volume 9, Basel: S. Karger AG, 1973, pp. 2-15.*

ischemia, it is logical to assume that the subendocardium of the left ventricle is the first area to be jeopardized (Figure 3-2). Since the earliest phase of ischemia produces irrever-sible elongation of myofibers, loss of contractility in the subendocardium appears first. This results in collapse of the intramyocardial microcirculation owing to bulging of the involved portion and affecting compression of the in-volved microcirculation (Figure 3-3).

The hemodynamic vise phenomenon can be clarified in the following fashion: Consider a series of straws, repre-senting the microcirculation, penetrating a sponge, repre-senting the myocardium. When the sponge is in a relaxed position, the straws will allow fluid to pass through the sponge with facility. By stretching the sponge, as occurs in the early phase of myocardial ischemia, the penetrating

LOSS OF CONTRACTILITY

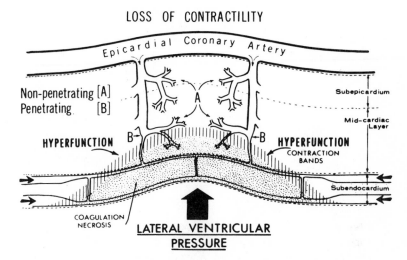

Figure 3-3. Schematic depicting the loss of contractility in the area where coagulation necrosis is taking place. With the loss of contractility in the subendocardium, the intramyocardial microcirculation is collapsed owing to bulging of the involved portion which compresses the involved microcirculation. Adjacent to the area of necrosis, there is a region of hyperfunctioning myocardial fibers. (A) Nonpenetrating coronary arteries. (B) Penetrating coronary arteries. Arrows demonstrate real and potential coronary flow. Reprinted with permission from Eliot, R.S.: Twentieth century stress and the subendocardium of the left ventricle. Transactions of the Association of Life Insurance Medical Directors of America, **57**:140, 1973.

straws (or microcirculatory vessels) are collapsed. Flow through the straws is significantly impeded. The increased resistance offered to flow from the epicardial vessels to the penetrating system of the microcirculation may occur in a similar fashion to that of the compressed straws in the stretched sponge. The absence of significant obstructive coronary disease would allow unimpeded collaterals to perfuse to the limits of the developing nontransmural infarction. In this setting, myocardial necrosis may be limited to

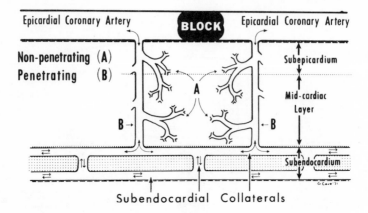

Figure 3-4. *Schematic depicting coronary blockage with normal collaterals. The block represents old or new blockage of a major epicardial coronary artery with adequate subendocardial collaterals preventing infarction. (A) Nonpenetrating coronary arteries. (B) Penetrating coronary arteries. Arrows demonstrate real and potential coronary flow. Reprinted with permission from Eliot, R.S. and Holsinger, J.W.: The pathophysiologic panorama of myocardial ischemia and infarction. In. J.H.K. Vogel (Ed.):* Myocardial Infarction: A New Look at an Old Subject, *Advances in Cardiology, Volume 9, Basel: S. Karger AG, 1973, pp. 2-15.*

the subendocardial region, resulting in a nontransmural myocardial infarction.

On the other hand, if a pre-existent obstruction exists in a major epicardial vessel, the microcirculatory stasis in concert with significant epicardial stenosis provides an ideal setting for coronary thrombosis at the point of maximum platelet adhesiveness. That point is known to be at the site of the longest and most narrowed luminal area of coronary atherosclerosis. Without extra- or intramyocardial circulatory pathways, massive myocardial infarction would seem inevitable (Figures 3-4 and 3-5).

The aforementioned hypothesis addresses itself to past and present data on pathophysiologic and morbid features of this disease. It will be recalled that nontransmural

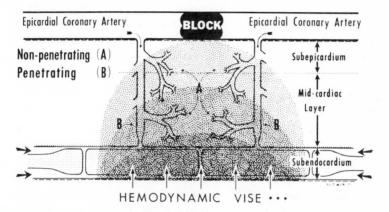

Figure 3-5. *Schematic depicting the progression of necrosis from the subendocardium to the subepicardium. Early necrotic changes in each layer progressively obliterate the collateral microcirculatory system. In the presence of epicardial blockage, subendocardial necrosis in an adjacent myocardial region will spread transmurally since all collateral circulation is destroyed with the advent of subendocardial infarction. (A) Nonpenetrating coronary arteries. (B) Penetrating coronary arteries. Arrows demonstrate real and potential coronary flow. Reprinted with permission from Eliot, R.S. and Holsinger, J.W.: The pathophysiologic panorama of myocardial ischemia and infarction. In J.H.K. Vogel (Ed.):* Myocardial Infarction: A New Look at an Old Subject, *Advances in Cardiology, Volume 9, Basel: S. Karger AG, 1973, pp. 2-15.*

myocardial infarction is usually associated with subtotal obstructive lesions, and that massive or transmural infarction is usually associated with one or more old complete obstruction(s) or severe old obstruction compromised by acute coronary thrombosis.[29,30] When viewed in this fashion, the loss of contractility is the primary domino in the development of typical myocardial infarction. Whether all the dominoes fall or not is dependent upon (1) the degree of stenosis of the epicardial coronary vessels, and (2) whether one or more key factors are sustained for a protracted period of time. After reaching the critical mass of necrosis with the resultant lowered pH, lysosomal degeneration can continue the myocardial necrotic process without external forces.

This pathophysiologic hypothesis lends itself to explaining the complications of myocardial infarction. First, arrhythmias are common in any and all forms of myocardial infarction. Second, the appendages of the subendocardium, namely the papillary muscles, have the same incidence of dysfunction and disruption in both forms of infarction owing to the same incidence of subendocardial necrosis — namely, 100 percent. Therefore, attendant mitral regurgitation also occurs equally. Rupture of the ventricular septum naturally is associated with transmural infarction in major coronary arterial obstruction, as ventricular aneurysm and external rupture of the heart are associated with pericardial tamponade. Mural thrombus and embolus remains the province of transmural myocardial infarction. Congestive heart failure with extensive transmural flail portions of the left ventricular wall (transmural) and cardiogenic shock is a more extreme example of the same phenomenon.

Certain complications of subendocardial infarction have caused it to be referred to as an incomplete infarction. Most difficult for the clinician to control is the persistent angina. Also, sudden death and reinfarction are most frequent in the first twelve months in nontransmural subendocardial myocardial infarctions. This hypothesis has practical implications. Among these are the consideration of patients for coronary bypass surgery.

Currently we offer coronary artery bypass surgery under the following circumstances: (1) individuals with angina refractory to medical management; (2) those with unstable angina; (3) critical lesions of the left coronary system; (4) complications of acute myocardial infraction, including cardiogenic shock; and (5) when significant coronary obstructive disease coexists with other cardiac lesions requiring operations such as valve replacement. Although unproven, the hypothesis discussed has been of great assistance to the author with regard to selecting individualized therapeutic measures, new or old.

PATHOPHYSIOLOGY OF SUDDEN DEATH

The definition of sudden unexpected coronary death adopted by the World Health Organization is death occurring within 24 hours of the onset of symptoms. Yet, in nearly half the reported cases, sudden deaths were "instantaneous", occurring within seconds or minutes of collapse.[31] Nearly two-thirds of the individuals so afflicted have no prior history of heart disease.[32] A number of investigators have considered sudden coronary death and acute myocardial infarction as different products of the same process, namely ischemic necrosis. They separate them only in a temporal sense. Acute myocardial infarction (AMI), of course, develops over a longer period of time than sudden coronary death (SCD).

It is important to mention certain key differences between these two conditions. For example, there is a much lower demonstrated incidence of acute occlusive coronary thrombi in victims of SCD than in AMI, as mentioned earlier.[12] In addition, fewer than one-third of patients dying within one hour of the onset of symptoms will exhibit an occlusive thrombus.[6,33] In one study, the incidence of occlusive thrombus was less than four percent when death occurred in less than 30 seconds.[31] It has already been observed that the longer the duration of cardiac symptoms prior to death, the greater the likelihood that an acute occlusive coronary thrombus will be present at necropsy.[7] The observation that an increased incidence of coronary thrombosis occurs with a longer duration of symptoms suggests that there is a different and distinct pathophysiologic mechanism for SCD than for AMI.

There are about 1,200 victims of sudden death per

day.[34] At least 25 percent have no prior recognized disease or stigmata.[34] The classic coronary risk factors are not selectively predictive and advanced coronary disease is not an exclusive requirement. Victims range in age from 20 years on up, with a median age of 69 years.[34] Sudden death is a leading cause of death in our society in people 20 to 64 years of age. In some, no evidence of myocardial infarction can be found by electrocardiography or serum enzyme elevation.[35] In this group, the incidence of sudden death was double that for survivors of AMI observed over a period of two years.[35] This implies that the mechanism for sudden death is frequently unrelated to ischemic mechanisms. Other factors, such as neurogenic hormones and catecholamines, may represent better explanations and thereby offer better therapeutic targets. It is of interest that in the studies of Ritchie et al[36] of 21 patients who survived episodes of ventricular fibrillation, thallium abnormalities (image at rest) were found in only 52 percent. This implies that those changes responsible for SCD may not involve typical myocardial necrosis or even ischemia uniformly. The frequent absence of acute occlusion has stimulated this work further.

Baroldi[37] has conducted highly detailed studies of 200 consecutive cases of sudden unexpected coronary death. It was determined that 76 percent of these cases demonstrated a unique focal form of myocardial necrosis referred to as coagulative myocytolysis. In another series, 81 percent of such victims demonstrated this lesion.[38] These lesions can also be found at the border of acute myocardial infarctions. Their presence in that location, however, is believed to be secondary to the infarction process and, therefore, to have a different significance.

Coagulative myocytolysis is a category of cell death which results from hyperfunctional overdrive. These myofibrillar lesions are distributed as widely scattered focal alterations which are located predominantly in the inner third of the left ventricle and are characterized by hypercontraction of the myofibrils (Figure 3-6). They appear as a

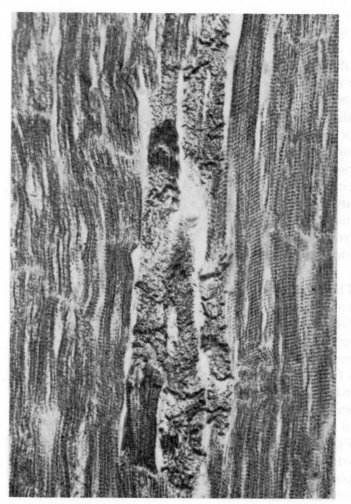

Figure 3-6. Coagulative myocytolysis resulting from hyperfunctional overdrive. This lesion is characterized by hypercontraction of the myofibrils. (PTAH × 524)

clump of sarcomeres that reveal an anomalous acidophilic crossband on standard H and E staining. These bands are surrounded on either end by a clearer area of myofibrillar rhexis. The lesions become visible very rapidly, possibly within minutes, and are easily detected by routine light microscopic techniques. In this form of necrosis, the early phase of myofibrillar damage is not accompanied by nuclear alterations. It is also distinguished from typical coagulation necrosis in that it does not involve polymorphonuclear leukocytic infiltration. The latter is the hallmark of coagulation necrosis, which automatically suggests an ischemic mechanism.[39,40] Experimental studies with electron microscopy reveal that there is an apparent breakdown of the anomalous contraction bands within about eight hours of their formation.[39] This breakdown results in vacuolated appearances leaving empty sarcolemmic tubes as the only evidence of the phenomena (Figure 3-7). Thus, coagulative myocytolysis is rapid in onset and in disappearance, leaving little detectable histologic evidence within 24 hours of its onset.

This hypercontracted form of myocardial necrosis appears to result from catecholamine overdrive. It frequently occurs in cases of pheochromocytoma, in selected forms of therapy such as bronchodilators (isoproterenol), appetite suppressants (amphetamines), intravenous infusions for shock (isoproterenol and other catecholamine-like agents), and in cases of increased sensitivity to treatment with MAO inhibitors. In our limited experience, it has often been observed in deaths related to a sudden emotional shock.

Experimental studies in our laboratory suggest that the majority of catecholamines, including epinephrine, norepinephrine and isoproterenol, are capable of causing extensive myocardial necrosis of the hyperfunctional variety, distinct from that of coagulation necrosis in myocardial infarction.[41] These observations provide additional evidence that this hyperfunctional form of necrosis may be induced by severe emotional stress and may precipitate SCD. Further evidence from our laboratory suggests that

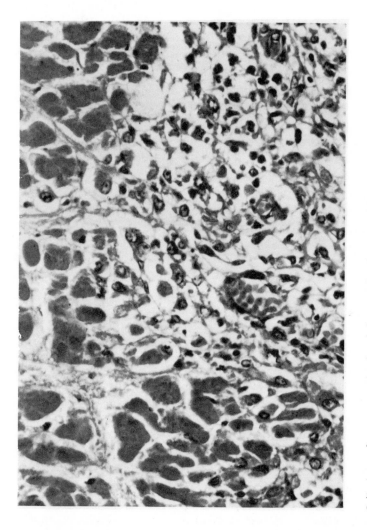

Figure 3-7. Anomalous contraction bands begin to be absorbed within about eight hours of formation resulting in a vacuolated appearance. These empty sarcolemmic tubes may be the only evidence of the phenomena. (H&E × 328)

these lesions, particularly the larger type, can be reduced either by lowering the dose of catecholamines or by pretreatment with propranolol.[41]

Precise pathophysiologic mechanisms relating catecholamines to other systems are presently being clarified, but further evidence is still required. Sympathomimetic overstimulation with resultant hypercontraction of the contractile filaments is readily apparent, but its effect on the heart and its role in cardiac death still need to be defined. These focal areas of necrosis probably reduce conduction velocity, thereby permitting re-entry phenomena. This is supported by the chaotic electrical storms leading to ventricular fibrillation. The latter is frequently observed during catecholamine infusion and appears in concert with the development of these lesions.

Aside from the well-known evidence that the sympathetic nervous system can contribute to, or indeed fundamentally induce, hyperfunctional necrosis, there is additional evidence that the sympathetic nervous system plays some key roles in the development of ventricular fibrillation. The prolonged QT interval syndrome or Jervell and Lange-Nielsen syndrome is sudden death (ventricular fibrillation) associated with congenital deafness and periods of syncope preceding the final event.[42] Romano[43] and Ward[44] have reported the same phenomenon without deafness in apparently normal individuals. There is some evidence that in certain patients dying of this syndrome, the conduction disturbances can be identified at the histopathologic level.[45] In others, however, nothing whatsoever is found despite careful search. Among the well-known electrocardiographic neurogenically induced changes are: increased QT interval, prominent Q waves, increased T waves, abnormally polar T waves or decreased ST segments or flattening of T waves. Ueda et al,[46] have shown a differential sympathetic response between the left and right stellate ganglia, and others have demonstrated that sympathetic outflow is variable from one part of the heart to another with focal involvement rather than a barrage of neurosympathetically discharged changes.[47] Stimulation, for example, of the ventrolateral nerve alters the refractory period of the posterior surface, whereas stimulation of the ventromedial nerve alters the refractory period of the anterior surface, and the recurrent nerve stimulation alters the same phenomenon near the ventricular septum. Recently, Schwartz et al[48] reported that ablating the right stellate ganglion will decrease the ventricular fibrillatory threshold, whereas ablation of the left stellate ganglion increases ventricular fibrillatory threshold. In such individuals, although cases are few in number, it appears likely that either ablation of the left stellate ganglion or beta blockade is the most effective means of preventing ventricular fibrillatory death owing to sympathetic nervous system outflow.

Both in the laboratory and in man, ventricular premature beats, or ventricular ectopy in general, are not uniform harbingers of ventricular fibrillation. The development of ventricular fibrillation in both settings may be spontaneous without electrocardiographic forewarning. In some instances, ventricular tachycardia unquestionably leads to ventricular fibrillation. However, the confounding aspect of ventricular ectopic beats is that they are ubiquitous.

It has been suggested by some that sudden death may be related to the embolization of cholesterol crystals from disrupted epicardial coronary atheromas.[49] It is hypothesized that sudden violent ventricular contraction may disrupt an atheroma and its associated vasa vasora, leading to hemorrhage into an atheromatous plaque. Extrusion of plaque into the lumen subsequently uncovers a nest of cholesterol crystals and atheromatous debris, permitting it to be washed downstream. In my experience, evidence for this hypothesis is meager, but may deserve further evaluation. Another popular hypothesis is the embolization of newly formed friable platelet thrombi from hypercoagulable epicardial coronary atheromatous sites. Evidence for reduced incidence of sudden death with sulfinpyrazone has lent preliminary enthusiasm to this hypothesis.[50]

The observation of coagulative myocytolysis in a rela-

tively large number of victims of sudden, unexpected cardiac death suggests that it may play a major role. It is possible that the number of lesions produced is directly related
to the likelihood of induced electrical or electrophysiologic
instability. Thus, the strength of the stimulus and its relationship to the myocardial response may be directly proportional to the number of lesions and, therefore, the likelihood of electrically-induced SCD.

A certain number of victims of SCD die without evidence of these lesions, without evidence of small vessel disease to the conduction system, or other indications of the
precise pathophysiologic mechanism. They may or may not
have associated chronic coronary artery disease of different
degrees. In these, it is proposed that some victims may have
acute myocardial ischemia, altered myocardial contractility,
electrical instability and ventricular arrhythmias. Therefore, an individual experiencing pain prior to sudden death
may belong to a different category of SCD.

Sudden Coronary Death on an Ischemic Basis

In view of the eight hour delay in the classic polymorphonuclear infiltration, investigators of sudden death
phenomena have sought earlier markers for coagulation
necrosis. In a certain number of individuals experiencing
sudden coronary death, the major histologic landmark is
elongated, thinned wavy fibers (Figure 3-8).[37] Similar features can be induced by ligation of the circumflex branch of
the left coronary system in a dog.[51] These features develop
within one hour. Despite the elongation of the fibers and,
more importantly, the nuclei, the striations of myofibrils
are maintained, so that nuclear changes and sarcoplasmic
eosinophilia are the earliest detectable light microscopic
changes.[52] With the assistance of the electron microscope,
one can observe the loss of glycogen accompanied by swelling, disruption and increased matrix density of mitochondria associated with nuclear chromatin margination or

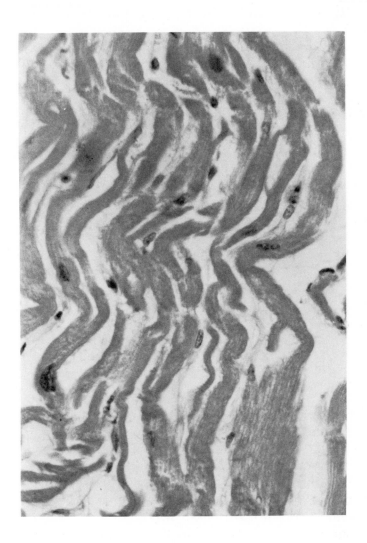

Figure 3-8. In certain victims of sudden coronary death, the major histologic landmark is elongated, thinned wavy fibers. The evidence for this is more substantial if there is elongation of nuclei on electron microscopic examination. (H&E × 328)

aggregation (Figure 3-9).[52] As might be expected, these lesions are most common in the subendocardium of the left ventricle. Despite their presence, the finding is not pathognomonic of ischemic necrosis. It falls into the category of "possible" only.

Among patients most frequently found to display elongated, thinned wavy fibers at necropsy are those in whom the usual clinical syndrome of myocardial infarction has developed but endured for less than six hours prior to death (isolated findings).[53] Elongated, thinned wavy fibers can be seen in areas subjacent to coagulative necrosis and acute myocardial infarction later on.[37] By contrast, those who have no pain prior to death and who die within a matter of seconds or minutes usually either display coagulative myocytolysis or fail to reveal any obvious histopathologic feature.[49,53]

Thus, the categories of myocardial necrosis associated with acute myocardial infarction or sudden coronary death involve two major categories:

1. Coagulation necrosis (AMI)
    a. established: polymorphonuclear leukocytic infiltration
    b. possible: elongated, thinned wavy fibers (early developing coagulation necrosis)
2. Coagulative myocytolysis (hyperfunctional)

The development of ischemic necrosis may be provoked by neurogenic hormonal mechanisms. The major factors are MVO_2, heart rate, myocardial contractile state, and wall tension. The product of the level of systolic pressure times the heart rate has formed a useful index (pressure-rate product) for the assessment of MVO_2 requirements. Any state contributing to high systolic pressure and rapid heart rate which is prolonged, severe and associated with a vulnerable coronary vascular system can logically lead to insufficient myocardial oxygenation. Emotional stress obviously fulfills the aforementioned prerequi-

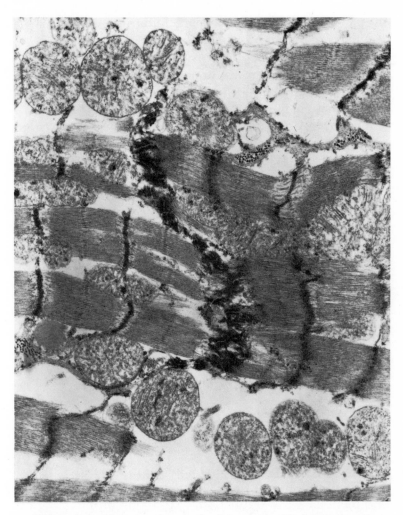

Figure 3-9. *Electron microscopic photograph of ischemic tissue in the dog myocardium one hour after ligation of the left circumflex coronary artery. There is a loss of glycogen accompanied by swelling and dense deposits of calcium in the mitochondria. This is distinct from that seen with anomalous contraction bands (see Figure 5). (× 13,250)*

sites and is a well-recognized precipitating factor in classic angina or acute myocardial infarction.

With the background provided, it can be proposed that under appropriate circumstances emotional stress can induce a state of visceral-vascular readiness. This may lead in either of two major pathophysiologic directions toward different forms of myocardial necrosis. The first is heralded by chest pain and represented by elongated, thinned wavy fibers; the second, on an even more acute basis and without forewarning, displays the histopathologic features of coagulative myocytolysis related to neurogenic hormonal overdrive. It is likely that admixtures of these two mechanisms exist.

Thus, in setting the stage for sudden coronary death, certain factors appear significant, singly or in concert. These include: (1) the state of the coronary vessels; (2) depletion of myocardial reserve with regard to factors yet undefined; (3) the duration of the physical or psychological stimulus; (4) the severity of the stimulus; and (5) the degree of individual physical and psychological resistance and resilience.

PATHOPHYSIOLOGY OF "ESSENTIAL" HYPERTENSION

The preoccupation with establishing a specific cause of hypertension, such as renal vascular disease, adrenocortical and medullary hyperfunction, coarctation of the aorta, eclampsia and others, has shown that only infrequently is an etiology discovered. It is generally understood that the cause of hypertension can be identified in less than 10 percent of cases. Furthermore, it is certainly not a rare disease. The most recent figures[54] point out that as of July 1977 there were 35 million definite hypertensives in the United States. Yet the "best estimates indicate that some 25 million additional persons have borderline hypertension."[54] If we

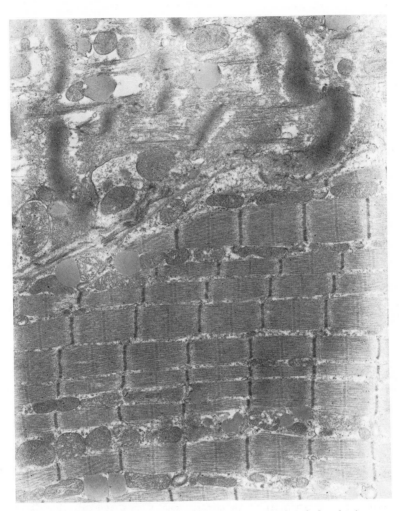

Figure 3-10. Electron microscopic photograph of developing anomalous contraction bands after infusion of isoproterenol (upper portion of photo). This is contrasted with the normal myofibrils in the lower portion of the photo. (× 9,275)

pick the figure of 140/90 mm Hg and apply that to the aforementioned figures, about 60 million Americans have blood pressure elevations at the time of this writing. Indeed, hypertension is so common as to make one wonder if something is being placed in the water supply. A remarkable contrast is to be found in the near total absence of hypertension in some primitive societies; yet immigrants from these groups to urban communities develop hypertension with equal or greater incidence and facility.[55]

As in most contemporary diseases of industrialized society, no single pathogenic mechanism can be identified. In 1949, Page[56] introduced the concept of a mosaic theory. Later, it was pointed out by Harris and Singer[57] that two primary pathways to hypertension may be involved on the basis of environmental factors.

Epidemiologic data point to an association between elevated systemic arterial blood pressure and socioenvironmental factors such as urban living, environmental threats, disruption of previous social patterns and environmental change or uncertainty. These life changes have been reflected in animal experiments. Work summarized by Mason[58] has shown that psychosocial stimuli can elicit either of two neuroendocrine responses. The first involves arousal of the pituitary adrenocortical system, and the second involves arousal of the sympathetic adrenal medullary system. Such arousals occur during confrontations between various members of a social group as they seek food, territory or mates. In the first (the alarm reaction), the sympathetic adrenal medullary system is called into play as agonist behavior is invoked in an attempt to maintain status and prevent threatened loss of esteem and/or related objects of attachment (Figure 3-11). In the second (playing dead), there is usually social interaction leading to downward displacement in the hierarchy which invokes stimulation of the pituitary adrenocortical system resulting in mental depression, decreased gonadotropin

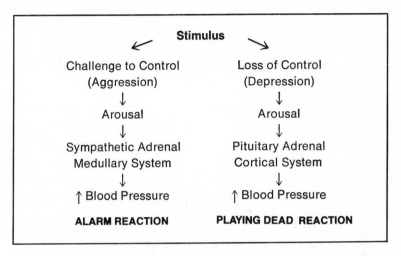

Figure 3-11. Two neuroendocrine pathways leading to hypertension. A stimulus which represents a challenge to control will lead to arousal and response through the sympathetic adrenal medullary system resulting in hypertension (the alarm reaction). A stimulus which represents loss of control will lead to arousal and response through the pituitary adrenal cortical system resulting in hypertension (the playing dead reaction). Adapted from Henry, J.P.: Understanding the early pathophysiology of essential hypertension. Geriatrics 31:59-72, 1976.

levels, enhanced vagal activity, gluconeogenesis and pepsin production.[59]

A classic demonstration of the latter is to be found in the studies of Von Holst,[60] who performed detailed experiments in adult male tree shrews. A subordinate animal was introduced to another male that was an experienced fighter. The dominant animal immediately attacked while the intruder submitted. The two animals were separated before injury could occur, but the subordinate was placed so that he could see the dominant animal without being attacked by him. The emotionally aroused subordinate lay still, watching the dominant animal's movement more than

90 percent of his waking time. The tail hair remained erect indicating a sustained sympathetic arousal. Within two to sixteen days, despite sufficient food and water intake, the subordinate animal fell into a coma and died. Elevated blood urea nitrogen and histologic evidence of renal failure pointed to acute renal vascular change as the cause of death.

In hypertension developed through the second pathway (playing dead reaction), there is an increase in ACTH activity associated with enhanced vagal activity. Increased gluconeogenesis, increased pepsin production, and decreased reticuloendothelial activity are found in conjunction with hypertension of this sort.

A variety of experiments have been conducted which confirm the validity of the repeated alarm reaction as a factor in sustained hypertension as outlined in the first pathway.[61,62] In this setting, there is an increase in blood pressure which is brought about by exaggerated sympathetic stimulation followed by an increase in cardiac output and an attendant increase in peripheral resistance. Associated with this change is an elevation in blood pressure, which may be transient unless the baroreceptor system becomes fixed due to a sustained alarm response. In addition, one finds an increase in fatty acids, glycogenolysis and catecholamine synthetic enzymes.

Effective management of labile hypertension which develops through the first pathway will lend itself to a variety of forms of nonpharmacologic management until such a time that the hypertension becomes less labile and the renal vascular changes become fixed. At that stage, pharmacologic management is the only option, owing to the irreversibility of vascular change.

Although the concept of a hypertensive personality remains ambiguous and lacks both experimental support and theoretical meaning, it is possible that the coping patterns of individuals vary on the basis of early experience as well as inherited potential. These may be the predominant contributors to the etiologic mosaic. For one individual there is a desire to maintain dominance and control. Such individuals may follow the first pathway to hypertension (alarm reaction). On the other hand, coping which involves a loss of control or the assumption of a subordinate position may be followed by hypertension of the second pathway (playing dead). Clinically, the former may be recognized as an individual who is aggressive, whereas the latter appears depressed.

It is an interesting clinical challenge to attempt to identify which pathway has been pursued toward the development of clinical hypertension in the labile phase of its development. Great insight into the life situation can be attained by the identification of the hypertensive pathway in question. Obviously, this will facilitate the planning of appropriate therapy.

It is apparent from the aforementioned paragraphs that hypertension may represent a maladjustment leading to a distinct disease process. Chronic hyperactive pressor responses to stimuli may thus be reflected in man, as they are in animals, by a temporary, and subsequently a more permanent, resetting of the baroreceptors. Thus, according to Shapiro,[63] hypertension is a disease of disordered regulation of homeostasis. In the early phase of the disease process, reversal by behavioral modification or reconditioning may be a valid form of therapy. Later, the vicious cycle of elevated blood pressure affecting the renin-angiotensin system develops with fixed vascular change. In this setting, inflexibility precludes successful control with the aforementioned techniques. Instead, pharmacologic intervention pointed at different pathophysiologic targets becomes essential.

Thus, it is apparent that hypertension best fits the mosaic theory of pathophysiology offered by Page,[56] in which two relatively distinct pathways can be outlined that represent individual coping maladjustments. Singularly or in concert with other factors, these pathways take into consideration the multiple influences attributed to psychosocial factors, catecholamines, neurogenic components, autoregulation, renal hypertension, sodium, reninangiotensin and mineralocorticoids. It has been pointed out that hypertension shares with other psychosomatic diseases specific disturbances or shifts in the bias of physiologic regulatory mechanisms.[64] If these become chronic, hypertension, too, may become chronic, fixed and less labile. Years of repeated psychosocial stimulation of the sympathetic adrenomedullary system (the alarm reaction) or of the pituitary adrenocrotical system (the playing dead reaction) can lead to hypertension associated, respectively, with either aggressive, behavior or passive, subordinate behavior.

Repeated arousal leads to structural vascular thickening and mechanically increased resistance. This may be associated with adrenomedullary and cortical hypertrophy which can intensify catecholamine, renin-angiotensin and adrenal cortical neuroendocrine responses. At this stage, the baroreceptors have been dulled by vessel wall changes and are less effective.[59]

Initially this deterioration is reversible. Furthermore, it would appear reversible by adjustment of the life situation employing nonpharmacologic techniques aimed at improving coping strategies, increasing physical activity and a variety of behavior modifying and reconditioning processes. Untreated, the condition may lead to permanent damage with fixed hypertension. One cannot underestimate the importance of psychosocial and neuroendocrine elements early, yet these become less significant in the late stages of hypertension.

To the clinician, the patient with labile hypertension may be displaying the most readily identifiable and objective indication of stress, thereby setting the stage for management employing the arts and techniques described in later chapters.

REFERENCES

1. Herrick, J.B.: Clinical features of sudden obstruction of the coronary arteries. *J.A.M.A.* **59**:2015-2020, 1912.

2. Branwood, A.W., and Montgomery, G.L.: Observations on the morbid anatomy of coronary artery disease. *Scottish Med. J.* **1**:367-375, 1956.

3. Spain, D.M., and Bradess, V.A.: Frequency of coronary thrombi as related to duration of survival from onset of acute fatal episodes of myocardial ischemia. *Circulation* **22**:816, 1960.

4. Roberts, W.C.: Coronary arteries in fatal acute myocardial infarction. *Circulation* **45**:215-230, 1972.

5. Baroldi, G., Radice, F., Schmid, G., and Leone, A.: Morphology of acute myocardial infarction in relation to coronary thrombosis. *Amer. Heart J.* **87**:65-75, 1974.

6. Haerem, J.W.: Mural platelet microthrombi and major acute lesions of main epicardial arteries in sudden coronary death. *Atherosclerosis* **19**:529, 1974.

7. Romo, M.: Factors related to sudden death in acute ischemic heart disease. *Acta Med. Scand.* Supplement 547:1, 1972.

8. Baroldi, G., and Scomazzoni, G.: *Coronary Circulation in the Normal and the Pathologic Heart,* Washington D.C.: U.S. Government Printing Office. 1967.

9. Erhardt, L.R., Lundman, T., and Mellstedt, H.: Incorporation of ^{125}I-labelled fibrinogen into coronary arterial thrombi in acute myocardial infarction in man. *Lancet* **1**:387, 1973.

10. Hackel, D.B., Estes, E.H., Walston, A., et al: Some problems concerning coronary artery occlusion and acute myocardial infarction. *Circulation* **40**: Supplement IV: 39, 1969.

11. Paterson, J.C.: Vascularization and hemorrhage of intima of arteriosclerotic arteries. *Arch. Pathol.* **22**:313, 1936.

12. Baroldi, G.: Acute coronary occlusion as a cause of myocardial infarct and sudden coronary heart death. *Amer. J. Cardiol.* **16**:859-880, 1965.

13. Enos, W., and Holmes, R.: Coronary disease among United States soldiers killed in action in Korea. *J.A.M.A* **152**:1090-1093, 1953.

14. Baroldi, G.: Unpublished data, 1977.
15. James, T.N.: Pathology of small coronary arteries. *Amer. J. Cardiol.* **20**:679-691, 1967.
16. Baroldi, G., and Manion, W.C.: Microcirculatory distur-bances and human myocardial infarction. *Amer. Heart J.* **74**:173-178, 1967.
17. Eliot, R.S., Baroldi, G., and Leone, A.: Necropsy studies in myocardial infarction with minimal or no coronary luminal reduction due to atherosclerosis. *Circulation* **49**:1127-1131, 1974.
18. Friedberg, C.K., and Horn, H.: Acute myocardial infarction not due to coronary artery occlusion. *J.A.M.A.* **112**:1675, 1939.
19. Gross, H., and Stenberg, W.H.: Myocardial infarction with-out significant lesions of coronary arteries. *Arch. Intern. Med.* **64**:249, 1939.
20. Oliva, P.B., Potts, D.E., and Pluss, R.G.: Coronary arterial spasm in Prinzmetal's variant form of angina. Documenta-tion of coronary arteriography. *New Eng. J. Med.* **288**:745-751, 1973.
21. Jennings, R.B., Warthan, W.B., and Zudyk, A.F.: Production of an area of homogeneous myocardial infarction in the dog. *Arch. Pathol.* **63**:580-585, 1975.
22. Maseri, A., Mimmo, R., Chierchia, S., et al: Coronary artery spasm as a cause of acute myocardial ischemia in man: *Chest* **68**:625, 1975.
23. Gensini, G.G.: *Coronary Arteriography,* Mt. Kisco, New York: Futura Publishing Co., 1975, p. 431.
24. Demeany, M.A., Tambe, A., and Zimmerman, H.A.: Coro-nary arterial spasm. *Dis. Chest* **53**:714, 1968.
25. O'Reilly, R.J., Spellberg, R.S., and King, T.W.: Recognition of proximal right coronary artery spasm during coronary arteriography. *Radiology* **95**:305, 1970.
26. Beck, H.G., and Suter, G.M.: Role of carbon monoxide in the causation of myocardial disease. *J.A.M.A.* **110**:1982, 1938.
27. Ehrich, W.E., Bellet, S., and Lewey, F.H.: Cardiac changes from CO poisoning. *Amer. J. Med. Sci.* **208**:511, 1944.

28. Barmeyer, J.: Physical activity and coronary collateral development. In V. Manninen and P.I. Halonen (Eds.): *Physical Activity and Coronary Heart Disease, Advances in Cardiology*, Vol. 18. Basel: S. Karger A.G., 1976, pp. 104–112.

29. Miller, R.D., Burchell, H.B., and Edwards, J.E.: Myocardial infarction with and without acute coronary occlusion. *Arch. Intern. Med.* **88**:597, 1951.

30. Chandler, A.B., Chapman, I., Erhardt, L.R., et al: Coronary thrombosis in myocardial infarction. Report of workshop on the role of coronary thrombosis in the pathogenesis of acute myocardial infarction. *Amer. J. Cardiol.* **34**:823, 1974.

31. Friedman, M., Manwaring, J.H., Rosenman, R.H., et al: Instantaneous and sudden deaths. Clinical and pathological differentiation in coronary artery disease. *J.A.M.A.* **225**:1319-1328, 1973.

32. Kuller, L., Perper, J., and Cooper, M.: Demographic characteristics and trends in arteriosclerotic heart disease mortality: Sudden death and myocardial infarction. *Circulation* **52**: Supplement III: 1-11, 1975.

33. Spain, D.M., and Bradess, V.A.: Sudden death from coronary heart disease. Survival time, frequency of thrombi and cigarette smoking. *Dis. Chest* **58**:107, 1970.

34. Lown, B.: Sudden cardiac death — The major challenge confronting contemporary cardiology. Opening Plenary Address, *27th Annual Scientific Session of the American College of Cardiology*, Anaheim, California, March 6, 1978.

35. Cobb, L.A., Jr.: Lessons learned from survivors of sudden cardiac death. *27th Annual Scientific Session of the American College of Cardiology*, Anaheim, California, March 6, 1978.

36. Ritchie, J.L., Hamilton, G.W., Trobaugh, G.B., et al: Myocardial imaging and radionuclide angiography in survivors of sudden cardiac death due to ventricular fibrillation: Preliminary report. *Amer. J. Cardiol.* **39**:852-857, 1977.

37. Baroldi, G.: Different types of myocardial necrosis in coronary heart disease. A pathophysiologic review of their functional significance. *Amer. Heart J.* **89**:742-752, 1975.

38. Lie, J.T., and Titus, J.L.: Pathology of the myocardium and the conduction system in sudden coronary death. *Circulation* **52**:41, 1975.

39. Bloom, S., and Cancilla, P.A.: Myocytolysis and mitochondrial calcification in rat myocardium after low doses of isoproterenol. *Amer. J. Pathol.* **54**:373-391, 1969.

40. Rona, G., Chappel, C.I., Balasy, T., and Caudry, R.: An infarct-like myocardial lesion and other toxic manifestations produced by isoproterenol in the rat. *Arch. Pathol.* **67**:443-455, 1959.

41. Eliot, R.S., Todd, G.L., Clayton, F.C., and Pieper, G.M.: Experimental catecholamine-induced acute myocardial necrosis. In V. Manninen and P.I. Halonen (Eds.): *Advances in Cardiology,* Volume 25, Basel: S. Karger AG, 1978, pp. 107-118.

42. Jervell, A., and Lange-Nielsen, F.: Congenital deaf-mutism, functional heart disease with prolongation of the QT interval, and sudden death. *Amer. Heart J.* **54**:59-68, 1957.

43. Romano, C., Gemme, G., and Pongiglione, R.: Aritmie cardiache rare dell'eta'pediatrica. *La Clinic Paediat.* **45**:656-683, 1963.

44. Ward, O.C.: A new familial cardiac syndrome in children. *J. Irish Med. Assoc.* **54**:103-106, 1964.

45. Fraser, G.R., Froggatt, P., and James, T.N.: Congenital deafness associated with electrocardiographic abnormalities, fainting attacks and sudden death. *Quart. J. Med.* **33**:361-385, 1964.

46. Ueda, H., Yanai, Y., Marao, S., et al: Electrocardiographic and vectorcardiographic changes produced by electrical stimulation of the cardiac nerves. *Japanese Heart J.* **5**:359, 1964.

47. Yanowitz, F., Preston, J.B., and Abildskov, J.A.: Functional distribution of right and left stellate innervation to the ventricles: Production of neurogenic electrocardiographic changes by unilateral alteration of sympathetic tone. *Circ. Res.* **18**:416-428, 1966.

48. Schwartz, P.J., Snebold, N.G., Brown, A.M.: Effects of unilateral cardiac sympathetic denervation on the ventricular fibrillation threshold. *Amer. J. Cardiol.* **37**:1034, 1976.

49. Baroldi, G.: Personal communication. April, 1978.

50. The Anthurane Reinfarction Trial Research Group: Sulfin-pyrazone in the prevention of cardiac death after myocardial infarction. The anthurane reinfarction trial. *New Eng. J. Med.* **298**:289-295, 1978.

51. Eliot, R.S., Clayton, F.C., Pieper, G.M., and Todd, G.L.: Influence of environmental stress on pathogenesis of sudden cardiac death. *Federation Proceedings* **36**:1719-1724, 1977.

52. Herdson, P.B., Somers, H.M., and Jennings, R.B.: A comparative study of the fine structure of normal and ischemic dog myocardium with special reference to early changes following temporary occlusion of a coronary artery. *Amer. J. Pathol.* **46**:367, 1965.

53. Eliot, R.S., Pieper, G.M., Clayton, F.C., and Todd, G.L.: Unpublished data, 1977.

54. Ward, G.W.: Info memo. National High Blood Pressure Education Program, National Heart, Lung, and Blood Institute, Department of Health, Education and Welfare. Number 13, May, 1978.

55. Gampel, M.B., Slome, C., Scotch, N., and Abramson, J.H.: Urbanization and hypertension among Zulu adults. *J. Chronic Dis.* **15**:67-70, 1972.

56. Page, I.H.: Pathogenesis of arterial hypertension. *J.A.M.A.* **140**:451-457, 1949.

57. Harris, R.E., and Singer, M.T.: Interaction of personality and stress in the pathogenesis of essential hypertension. In J.E. Wood (Ed.): *Hypertension. Neural Control of Arterial Pressure. Proceedings of the Council on High Blood Pressure Research*, Vol. 16, New York: American Heart Association, 1968.

58. Mason, J.W.: A review of psychoendocrine research on the pituitary-adrenal cortical system. *Psychosomatic Med.* **30**:576-607, 1968.

59. Henry, J.P.: Understanding the early pathophysiology of essential hypertension. *Geriatrics* **31**:59-72, 1976.

60. Von Holst, D.: Renal failure as the cause of death in tupaia belangeri (tree shrews) exposed to persistent social stress. *J. Comprehensive Physiol.* **78**:236, 1972.

61. Henry, J.P., Ely, D.L., and Stephens, P.M.: Changes in catecholamine-controlling enzymes in response to psychosocial activation of the defence and alarm reactions. In *Physiology, Emotion and Psychosomatic Illness, Ciba Foundation Symposium 8*. Amsterdam: Associated Scientific Publishers, 1972, pp. 225–251.

62. Herd, J.A., Morse, W.H., Kelleher, R.T., and Jones, L.G.: Arterial hypertension in the squirrel monkey during behavioral experiments. *Amer. J. Physiol.* **217**:24-29, 1969.

63. Shapiro, A.P.: Behavioral approach to the study of cardiovascular disease in man. In A. Zanchetti (Ed.): *Neural and Psychological Mechanisms in Cardiovascular Disease*, Milan: Il Ponte, 1972, pp. 75-83.

64. Weiner, H.: Are "psychosomatic" diseases diseases of regulation? *Psychosomatic Med.* **37**:289, 1975.

CHAPTER 4

DIAGNOSTIC TOOLS

The practical application of the role of stress in cardiovascular and other diseases has been delayed by the lack of objective indices. An index can only be of practical value if it has proven prognostic significance. The assessment of success for any diagnostic test is based upon its sensitivity, specificity and selectivity. Sensitivity is the extent to which patients who truly manifest a disease are so classified, whereas specificity is the extent to which patients without the disease are correctly classified.[1] On the other hand, the selectivity of a test is the extent to which it differentiates the disease in question from all others. For a disease as common as coronary heart disease, almost any common component of an industrialized society will display some sensitivity. Contemporary correlations, both rational and bizarre, have been drawn with statistical significance between a variety of environmental and behavioral circumstances and the likelihood of coronary heart disease or sudden coronary death.

Frequently we are told that a given factor or index doubles the likelihood of a coronary event. Put into realistic clinical perspective, this may mean the difference between one and two coronary events per 100 patients seen by an individual physician. It is truly the impossible dream for the clinician to identify the small number of "at risk" patients from the huge number who are less endangered that year. Sensitivity and selectivity are statistical goals for epidemiologists, but are of trivial value for the clinician facing individual cases. Indeed, given any risk, it is impossible to predict counteracting forces on a constitutional or environmental basis.

Although imperfect, many new psychological tools offer us some perspective and insight regarding our patients. For the time being, we may have to rely on such ephemeral attributes as our clinical acumen to select the patient at greatest risk when psychological tests identify potential danger. The review of current diagnostic tools in this chapter includes a variety of testing methods related only within the goals and objectives of this text.

PSYCHOLOGICAL TOOLS

The Jenkins Activity Survey

In an attempt to quantify type A and type B behavior, Jenkins[2] has assembled a written questionnaire to substitute for the less reproducible subjective interview technique of Rosenman and Friedman. Critics of the test suggest that it does not include the hostility quotient or the facility with which an individual is aroused, believed by Rosenman and Friedman to be a fundamental component of the type A behavior pattern. According to Jenkins, "It is premature to use the Activity Survey in counseling or treating patients because it misclassifies too many individuals in terms of their future chances of developing clinical disease."[3] At the present time, the test is distributed for research purposes only. Differentiation between type A and type B individuals employing the Jenkins Activity Survey scores agrees 73% with the assessment by the structured interview.[4] Others who have attempted to utilize either the type A interview or the Jenkins Activity Scale are frequently troubled by the random nature of the associations.

In fairness, it must be said that there is a strong impression in the clinical community that the type A behavior pattern is a contributor to coronary heart disease. What is lacking is a truly objective, reliable assessment of this characteristic, as well as a method of determining the individual counterbalancing resources available from a constitutional or environmental standpoint. In some settings, there may be genuine rewards and psychological support for type A behavior. An individual so rewarded may be less stressed, less frustrated and at normal risk. Of the protective resources, the resilience and coping capacity of the individual appear to be the most critical. However, objective quantitation of these resources is not possible at present. It is probable that the multifactorial "web of causation" in coronary heart disease limits the significance of any single risk factor. For example, type A individuals exhibit 1.7 to 4.5 times the rate of coronary heart disease as type B individuals.[5] Were it possible to isolate this risk, it would be equal to the risk of neglecting seat belts throughout one's driving career. The Western Collaborative Group Study (WCGS) demonstrated type A behavior to have predictive capability prospectively for large populations.[6] Its value in the individual case remains a goal rather than a conclusion.

The Recent Life Change Questionnaire (RLCQ)

Holmes and Rahe[7] have attempted to define the stresses of life change by employing a numerical index; the index includes such life changes as death of a spouse, trouble with the boss, divorce, assumption of a large mortgage and so forth. Initially, the indices incorporated weighted values for different events. For example, the death of a spouse was weighted several times as significant as a dog bite. These weighted values fail to take into consideration the individual life situation and perception of the person experiencing the life event, and for that reason they lack selective capability. Here again, the question of coping reserve arises.

Earlier in this text it was noted that modern members of industrialized society experience in one year one thousand times the number of events experienced by those who lived a century ago. The hypothesis of Holmes and Rahe implies that one's psychological circuits can become overloaded. When overloading with input and decision-making occurs to the extent that stress and its resultant alarm reaction are suspended and prolonged, the overloading ultimately predisposes certain individuals to coronary heart disease as well as other major illnesses. Retrospective studies have indicated that such illnesses frequently correlate with high life change indices.[8-10] Prospective studies, however, have been less selective and, therefore, less successful in the individual case.[11-13] Again, there may be failure of the test to define individual constitutional or environmental counterforces of resilience.

The predictive capability of the RLCQ also depends upon the time frame or series of time frames being assessed. If one examines the entire year prior to an event, it may not be as valuable as noting the build up of events from four to six months prior to the stress-induced situation.

One of the values of the questionnaire is that it explores various portions of a person's life, such as health, work, family, personal, social and financial circumstances. Each may assist the physician in identifying problem areas where individual counseling can be of benefit. Awareness of these factors may not prevent death or infarction, but when properly utilized by the physician may indicate clinical targets for improving the quality of life. Reduction of the number of events, in my experience, has been very important in controlling anxiety and stress from overloaded circuits. The result has been an improved quality of life for many of my patients. For example, why plan a dental appointment, an argument with the boss, and a visit from your mother-in-law on the same rainy Tuesday?

An obvious limitation of the RLCQ is that it does not account for individual perception of the event, unique resources for solution and other factors of resilience. For example, an individual whose profession requires frequent geographic change might well be under less stress from a change in location than an individual who had been employed in the same place geographically for a 25 year period. Also, the examination cannot selectively predict which individuals will or won't develop coronary heart disease. It is unlikely that any single test will develop as an absolute predictor of coronary or no coronary heart disease.

A further problem with any questionnaire is that the responses may not always be an accurate reflection of the individual's life. The response may depict hope rather than reality. The person may, for example, want a life change to be the cause of his problems; therefore, his answers may reflect a distorted perception, thereby introducing error. When used cautiously, this test again may have clinical usefulness as a guide. While its predictive limitations are clear, further investigation will be required to determine its ultimate role in clinical medicine.

The Cattell Anxiety Scale

Sometimes it is useful to objectively measure the level of patient anxiety which might be exacerbating the patient's medical condition. The Cattell Anxiety Scale is quite acceptable for this purpose. It is also useful in assessing the treatment effects of particular drugs or behavioral manipulations, such as exercise or relaxation techniques. This scale has been used extensively and has been tested for validity and reliability.[14-16] It is limited in that it measures only anxiety states. As a measurement of stress, it focuses only upon this sphere. However, when the physician desires to test the effectiveness of any method in reducing anxiety, the Cattell Scale is a useful consideration.

The Zung Depression Index

The Zung Depression Index is a brief-self-administered depression measurement which has been used extensively in psychiatric research.[17] It is considered to be a valid measure of depressive symptomatology.[18,19] In a patient depicting depression, it may be of use to the clinician desiring an index of change. It will be recalled, however, that it measures only the parameters of depression, and not other considerations. Such surveys often require consultation for appropriate interpretation.

The Leighton Health Opinion Survey

The Leighton Health Opinion Survey measures psychoneuroticism and is useful as a general measure of psychiatric "caseness".[20] The latter term implies the likelihood that an individual tested would develop overt psychiatric symptomatology in the future. Its predictive capability is reasonably accurate, yet interpretation from one research group to another varies.[21]

The Minnesota Multiphasic Personality Inventory (MMPI)

Undoubtedly the most thoroughly evaluated, extensively implemented and validated study to assess psychological parameters is the Minnesota Multiphasic Personality Inventory (MMPI). It is capable of assessing traits that are commonly characteristic of disabling psychological abnormality.[22] It covers a wide variety of content, ranging from health to social attitudes. Five hundred fifty items are assessed in the self-administered examination. It has been used successfully in differentiating individuals who are normal from those who have neuroses or from those who have psychoses. This can frequently be of value to the clinician, and also offers the opportunity to identify psychological areas of particular importance in a given patient.

Its limitations are that it is time consuming (there are five hundred fifty items) and that its interpretation requires extensive clinical training and experience. Little has been done with the MMPI to correlate positive findings with the predictive potential for hypertension or coronary heart disease.

PHYSIOLOGICAL AND BIOCHEMICAL TOOLS

Catecholamine Assay

In view of the well-known association between the autonomic nervous system (in particular the sympathetic nervous system) and the cardiovascular response to stress, it is not surprising that catecholamines have been considered an appropriate measurement for stress. Indeed, serum or urinary catecholamine levels have been offered as an objective measure of the degree of stress experienced in an individual case. Unfortunately, these levels may be affected by variables other than adrenergic function. For example, alterations of neuronal reuptake and storage, differences in tissue metabolism and renal clearance can confound their use in clinical medicine.[23] To the present time, the use of catecholamines in determining the level of stress, the effects of therapy, or the success of prevention remains in the investigative stage.

Serum Dopamine Beta Hydroxylase (DBH)

Serum dopamine beta hydroxylase (DBH) is an enzyme that converts dopamine to norepinephrine within the sympathetic nervous system. There is no established pathway of excretion. It appears to have a longer half-life than catecholamines themselves. It has been proposed that DBH activity provides an index of sympathetic nervous system function.[24] As such, it may offer a better guide to chronic adrenergic activity than catecholamine levels. This analysis appears to be a more valid option for future clinical implementation.

Electrocardiogram

Schiffer and colleagues[25] demonstrated that an ego-threatening quiz given during electrocardiographic monitoring over a period of 12 minutes elicited significantly larger elevations in heart rate and blood pressure among those patients who exhibited objective signs of ischemic heart disease (i.e., angina). Indeed, the predictive capability of the emotional test correlated well with positive treadmill testing. The correlation was high (r = 0.63) between exercise and emotional stress situations for the level of ST segment depression. In a similar study with tighter experimental controls, Sime[26] reported no significant difference in heart rate or blood pressure response to the ego-threatening quiz between post-infarct patients and matched control subjects without disease. However, there was a significant difference between the sedentary type A patients and the active exercising type B patients. The latter group showed significantly lower heart rate and blood pressure responses.

Another useful psychological stress is to ask the patient to recall his most painful emotional experience while he is attached to an electrocardiographic monitoring device. Lown[27] has found this useful in detecting and controlling untoward ventricular ectopic rhythms. Recognizing that the population sample size in these studies was relatively small and the experience equally small, this form of evaluation appears to be efficacious for clinicians who are interested in documenting the electrophysiological response to emotional stress. In my experience, it is often useful to interview patients with one eye on the patient and the other eye on the monitor.

Galvanic Skin Responses

Under conditions of emotional stress and the associated alarm reaction, the skin resistance to voltage conductance is lower due to the presecretory activity of the membranes of the sweat gland cells.[28] Accordingly, it appears to be a valid means of detecting physiologic response to symbolic psychological input. This technique may lead to further understanding of the interrelationship between physiologic arousal and the defensive responses of the individual. It offers the potential for measuring autonomic arousal.

Peripheral Blood Flow

Plethysmography of the forearm has been frequently used as a measure of peripheral blood flow. The measurement is valuable in that it is highly specific for emotional stress. Changes in peripheral blood flow were observed in situations of emotional stress, specifically mental arithmetic and a word/color frustration task.[29] By contrast, little or no change in response was observed during physical stressors, such as pain and hot or cold water immersion in the contralateral arm.[30] Forearm blood flow increases occur only when a patient perceives a situation to be threatening or where mental concentration and problem-solving is required under scrutiny with the threat of criticism.[31] Similar observations were made by Williams,[32] who demonstrated that some of the individual differences in forearm blood flow response to a mental concentration task could be accounted for by personality characteristics.

SUBJECTIVE TOOLS

Fundamental to the subjective testing of individuals is the question of who should administer the tests. Should it be the physician in charge, a psychiatrist or psychologist? It is my view that the majority of patients can be interviewed by the physician himself. In each instance, it is a matter of the orientation of the physician — his background, goals of practice, his available resources, and interests.

At the present time, the reward systems in medicine are not geared toward lengthy consultations with patients. There is even a negative incentive for thorough searching interviews aimed at reconstructing or preventing cardiovascular catastrophe. While most of the material rewards focus on a variety of technical measurements and interventions, it has been my experience that the personal and professional rewards for thoroughly interviewing patients are most gratifying. Equally, I have found patients quite willing to spend the time and the money to develop awareness, insight, and methods for improving the quality of their lives. Also, adherence to therapeutic regimens is more likely with this approach.

FUTURE CONSIDERATIONS

Each of the aforementioned tests must be considered within its limitations. Since we remain unable to isolate and reliably predict individuals at risk rather than populations at risk, major efforts must be directed toward defining individual sensitivity and selectivity to the effects of lifestyle, behavior and perception.

Researchers must work toward the goal of accuracy, precision and reproducibility. It is the view of my colleagues and I that the development of such techniques can be facilitated by employing the concept of the elastic modulus. This concept involves the recognition that a force applied to an object does work against it and may stretch it in an elastic fashion. The extent to which it stretches, the speed with which it stretches, the duration of time that it remains stretched, the rapidity with which it returns to normal or the inability to return to normal are each parameters of elastic measurement which can apply to human physiology. Consider the possibility that two individuals are asked the same question while they are monitored for changes in electrocardiogram, respiratory rate, blood pressure, and skin resistance. Their objective responses to a written question or their oral responses to a subjective question may be identical. Yet their physiologic responses may be completely disparate. In one instance, an increase in heart rate, without accompanying blood pressure and skin resistance changes, could quickly return to normal. In the other instance, heart rate, blood pressure, and skin resistance might move several standard deviations from normal, be slow to return or fail to return to normal after a given period of time. Knowledge that there is an incongruity between the verbal or written response and the physiologic response, as well as knowledge of the degree of change from normal, may allow one to put numbers on such sociobiologic events. Furthermore, techniques of this variety are useful in clinical medicine as they employ methods that are common in clinical practice and do not require elaborate equipment or undue expense.

Armed with the knowledge that a patient is overreactive to some parameters of his health, his social activities, his family, his job, and so forth, the physician can be more precise in placing priorities for intervention.

At this writing, in the Stress Physiology Laboratory of the University of Nebraska, investigations are under way to unravel the practical capabilities of some of these diagnostic tools.

REFERENCES

1. MacMahon, B., and Pugh, T.F.: *Epidemiology: Principles and Methods.* Boston: Little, Brown and Co., 1970.
2. Jenkins, C.D., Rosenman, R.H., and Friedman, M.: Development of an objective psychological test for the determination of the coronary-prone behavior pattern in employed men. *J. Chronic Dis.* **20**:371-379, 1967.
3. Jenkins, C.D.: Personal communication, 1976.
4. Jenkins, C.D., Zyzanski, S.J., and Rosenman, R.H.: Progress

toward validation of a computer-scored test for the Type A coronary-prone behavior pattern. *Psychosomatic Med.* **33**:193, 1971.

5. Jenkins, C.D.: The coronary-prone personality. In W.D. Gentry and R.B. Williams (Eds.): *Psychological Aspects of Myocardial Infarction and Coronary Care.* St. Louis: C.V. Mosby Co., 1975, pp. 5-23.

6. Rosenman, R.H., Brand, R.J., Jenkins, C.D., et al: Coronary heart disease in the Western Collaborative Group Study. Final follow-up experience of 8½ years. *J.A.M.A.* **233**:872-877, 1975.

7. Holmes, T.H., and Rahe, R.H.: The social readjustment rating scale. *J. Psychosomatic Res.* **11**:213-218, 1967.

8. Rahe, R.H., Romo, M., Bennett, L., and Siltanen, P.: Subjects' recent life changes, myocardial infarction and abrupt coronary death. *Arch. Intern. Med.* **133**:221-228, 1974.

9. Rahe, R.H., Arajarvi, H., Arajarvi, S., et al: Recent life changes and coronary heart disease in East versus West Finland. *J. Psychosomatic Res.* **20**:431-437, 1976.

10. Rahe, R.H.: Stress and strain in coronary heart disease. *J. South Carolina Med. Assoc.* (Supplement) **72**:7-14, 1976.

11. Goldberg, E.L., and Comstock, G.W.: Life events and subsequent illness. *Amer. J. Epidemiol.* **104**:146-158, 1976.

12. Rahe, R.H.: The pathway between subjects' recent life changes and their near-future illness reports: Representative results and methodological issues. In B.S. Dohrenwend and B.P. Dohrenwend (Eds.): *Stressful Life Events.* New York: John Wiley and Sons, 1974, pp.73–86.

13. Holmes, T.S.: Adaptive behavior and health change. Medical thesis, University of Washington, Seattle, 1970.

14. Bendig, A.W.: Comparative reliability of Cattell's "covert" and "overt" items as measures of the anxiety factor. *J. General Psychology* **69**:175-179, 1963.

15. Bendig, A.W.: The factorial validity of items on the IPAT anxiety scale. *J. Consulting Psychology* **24**:374, 1960.

16. Bendig, A.W.: College norms for and concurrent validity of Cattell's IPAT anxiety scale. *Psychology Newsletter N.Y.U.* **10**:263-267, 1959.

17. Zung, W.W.: A self-rating depression scale. *Arch. General Psychiatry* **12**:63-70, 1965.
18. Zung, W.W., Richards, C.B., and Short, M.J.: Self-rating depression scale in an outpatient clinic. Further validation of the SDS. *Arch. General Psychiatry* **13**:508-515, 1965.
19. Marone, J., and Lubin, B.: Relationship between set 2 of the depression adjective check lists (DACL) and Zung self-rating depression scale (SDS). *Psychology Reports* **22**:233-234, 1968.
20. Leighton, D.C., Harding, J.S., Macklin, D.G., et al: *The Character of Danger.* New York: Basic Books, 1963, p. 121.
21. Tousignant, M., Denis, G., and Lachapelle, R.: Some considerations concerning the validity and use of the health opinion survey. *J. Health & Social Behavior* **15**:241-252, 1974.
22. Anastasi, A.: *Psychological Testing.* New York: Macmillan, 1954.
23. Stone, R.A., and DeLeo, J: Psychotherapeutic control of hypertension. *New Eng. J. Med.* **294**:80-84, 1976.
24. Silbergeld, S., Manderscheid, R.W., O'Neill, P.H., et al: Changes in serum dopamine-β-hydroxylase activity during group psychotherapy. *Psychosomatic Med.* **37**:352-367, 1975.
25. Schiffer, F., Hartley, L.H., Schulman, C.L., and Abelmann, W.H.: The quiz electrocardiogram: A new diagnostic and research technique for evaluating the relation between emotional stress and ischemic heart disease. *Amer. J. Cardiol.* **37**:41-47, 1976.
26. Sime, W.E.: Electrocardiogram and blood pressure responses to emotional stress (quiz interview) in post-infarct cardiac patients and matched control subjects. Unpublished, 1978.
27. Lown, B., Verrier, R.L., and Rabinowitz, S.H.: Neural and psychologic mechanisms and the problem of sudden cardiac death. *Amer. J. Cardiol.* **39**:890-902, 1977.
28. Lader, M.: Psychophysiological parameters and methods. In L. Levi (Ed.): *Emotions – Their Parameters and Measurement.* New York: Raven Press, 1975, pp. 341-365.
29. Stroop, J.R.: Interference in serial verbal reactions. *J. Experimental Psychology* **18**:643-661, 1935.
30. Konzett, H., and Strieder, K.: Differentiation of stress stimuli

by measuring forearm blood flow. *Federation Proceedings* **29**:741, 1970 (abstract 2801).

31. Konzett, H.: Cardiovascular parameters and methods of measuring emotions. In L. Levi (Ed.): *Emotions — Their Parameters and Measurement.* New York: Raven Press, 1975, pp. 369-378.

32. Williams, R.B., Jr., Poon, L.W., and Burdette, L.J.: Locus of control and vasomotor response to sensory processing. *Psychosomatic Med.* **39**:127, 1977.

CHAPTER 5

BEHAVIORAL THERAPIES

The human race has had to avoid certain catastrophes in order to survive. Among today's highest risks are ecological, technological, nuclear and political disasters. Optimistically, preventive measures are available. If we are to avoid these disasters, yet another critical factor challenges future planners: can humans learn to cope with the required rapid changes? Political scientists use the term "impact point" to indicate a projected date when human life and the environment become incompatible.

Anthropologists have identified the effect of such impact points during evolution. Leakey,[1] for example, is increasingly concerned about overpopulation, environmental abuses and the depletion of natural resources, fearing that man may be unable to cope biologically. These factors could be the basis for the first "impact point", projected to be the year 2000. Obviously, genetic selection or change is too leisurely to assure survival in a rapidly changing, often hostile environment. According to Leakey, "People feel that we are here by predestination and that because we are humans we will be able to survive even if we make mistakes".[1] Because there is a tendency to disregard the fact that humans are living organisms, Leakey has expressed further concern: "There have been thousands of living organisms of which a very high percentage has become extinct. There is nothing, at the moment, to suggest that we are not part of the same pattern." He notes, however, that there is a major difference: Man is the only organism with power to reflect on his past and future. The power to reflect "is what makes us able to plan our future in such a way as to

85

avoid what seems inevitable".[1] Whether we can learn to change rapidly enough is the critical question in the view of many.

One has only to reflect upon the past decade to note the rapid changes in our environment. The increasing complexity of the health professions is but one example, all too familiar to the reader. Our view of the future is myopic and guarded. There are too many unpredictable factors beyond individual, governmental or international control. It thus remains a complex political, sociological, medical and ethical question to determine optimal behavioral modification for these times.

Yet it is not the purpose or responsibility of physicians to point the direction of society, its corporations' goals or its politics. These functions remain the responsibility of statesmen and business leaders, and require the best of their collective wisdom and foresight. Obviously there are, and will be, mistakes emanating from the most thoughtful and sage of these leaders and the cultures of the future. Therefore, the ability to cope in today's terms looms essential both now and in the future.

In medical practice, new therapeutic measures of this type require ethical considerations to be incorporated in the guidelines for behavioral therapies. For example, if we produce an individual who is modified to the extent that he has lost his relevance or ability to function appropriately in his environment and society, we have contributed not only to the demise of the individual, but to the demise of his society as well. History has taught us that behavioral manipulation for large masses of people can itself lead to a myriad of national and international disasters (i.e., Nazi Germany).

Modification of behavior, then, must consider the individual himself, his potential, and what his role is in a changing society, in order that it may meet optimal preventive or therapeutic medical needs. In industrialized nations, coronary-prone behavior is a major potential therapeutic

target. It is my contention that skilled therapeutic modification of this behavior belongs in informed clinical settings
and not in cults. Although this is an area unfamiliar to the
medical practitioner, it appears to offer new dimensions to
his effectiveness in patient management. This chapter provides a background for the interested clinician, in order
that he may select some of the more realistic and useful
behavioral therapies for practical application to patients
with recognized needs.

To better meet the totality of human needs, the relationship between mind and body must be acknowledged
and better understood. The new field of behavioral
medicine creates such a forum through the integration of
many disciplines into a common framework to provide a
more comprehensive and balanced approach to human
health and disease.

CLINICAL BACKGROUND

In clinical cardiology, as in other areas of medicine,
there are a large number of patients who are experiencing
varying degrees of problems in living. One portion of this
group may be characterized as "worried but well", that is,
individuals who are basically emotionally mature and who
function well in most areas of their private and public lives.
Yet, they complain about such things as job pressures,
inability to relax, and being easily upset. When properly
motivated, these individuals can, on their own or with minimal, even non-professional help, learn to cope better. In
many of these cases, the problem usually results from a
simple lack of information on how to deal with certain difficulties.

A portion of these patients has more serious emotional
and behavioral problems. Since most of the problems
center in the area of close interpersonal relationships (viz,
the family), they are often not readily apparent. Typical

problems here are the inability to communicate feelings, difficulty in self-assertion, conflicts with children, and a variety of sexual dysfunctions. These problems are best managed by formal counseling or psychotherapy.

It is to be stressed that what distinguishes the cardiovascular patients from other medical patients or from the population in general is the nature of their physical illness rather than their emotional or behavioral characteristics. Undoubtedly, these physical problems contribute to the behavioral characteristics as well as perhaps resulting from them. In addition, it has been proposed that the so-called coronary-prone behavior is a significant risk factor itself.

The importance of behavioral, as well as biomedical, factors in cardiovascular disorders has prompted me to invite my colleague in behavioral psychology, Dr. Hermann Witte, to join me in the writing of this chapter. His background includes five years of experience in behavioral therapy with cardiac patients at a leading rehabilitation clinic in West Germany. Our combined interest, experience and background should provide a useful dialogue for developing current and practical guidelines for the implementation of this important therapeutic method.

The reader must avoid confusing behavioral therapy with psychoanalysis. The latter is often viewed as a form of psychological and emotional treatment in which the patient goes to a psychiatrist two or three times a week, lies down on a couch beneath a picture of Freud, and free-associates at length about various things which the analyst then explores for hidden sexual meaning. The focus is upon historical happenings, notably childhood experiences, as determinants for present problems. The examination and resolution of Oedipal complexes, castration fears, and related rumblings in the id are the primary targets of this form of therapy, which may continue for many years.

In contrast, behavioral therapy is a very different endeavor. As a psychotherapeutic school, it began nearly three decades ago, yet it has only recently become popular. Since it offers new therapeutic dimensions, it seems important that this body of information be made available for use in everyday clinical settings. To our contemporaries in medicine, this field can be viewed as a sublimated quantum leap from the "toilet training" approach of the classical psychoanalytic era. It utilizes some unique and reasonably sensible approaches to dealing with the problems of living and their relationship to health and disease.

Behavioral therapy is a scientific discipline based upon a great deal of experimental and clinical research into the nature of learning. What has emerged from this research is the knowledge that human behavior and behavioral change are associated with one or more of four basic concepts of learning:

1. *Conditioning:* Emotional, autonomic, and behavioral reactions occur in response to stimuli with which they have been repeatedly paired or associated.

2. *Effect:* Responses are shaped, and ultimately strengthened or weakened, on the basis of the effects or the consequences which they produce.

3. *Modeling:* Organisms, and especially human beings, copy the behavior of others.

4. *Cognition:* Thoughts which are immediately attached to perceptions determine the resultant emotional and behavioral responses and not the perceptions themselves.

The behavioral concept assumes that all behavior is a product of perception, mediated by the thought process and various emotional and autonomic responses. Put another way, behavior is the final link in a stimulus-coping-response chain. An understanding of this linkage within the framework of the aforementioned concepts offers the clinician an opportunity to analyze the chain and detect the faulty link. It can then be replaced with another link, permitting more problem-free behavior.

The great value of the behavioral model is that it emphasizes current and ongoing factors influencing behavior. Previously, the doctrine of Freud argued that most behavior was unalterably fixed in early childhood. Although the importance of childhood influences on an individual's problems is not denied, behavioral therapy does not dwell upon them to the same degree as heretofore. Instead, attention is directed to the immediate precipitants and the immediate consequences of behavior as the critical factors. For example, a patient might complain that he has always been, and continues to be, exploited. For the purpose of stopping that exploitation, it is far more important to point out that he is passive and non-assertive than to explore the original whens and whys of the problem. Passive or non-assertive behaviors can be demonstrated to invite and maintain exploitation. Becoming appropriately assertive can diminish or eliminate the problem. The therapist conveys the belief to the patient that his problems are the product of faulty learning and that unlearning as well as new learning is possible. The emphasis is thereby placed on the individual's coping resources. Stated otherwise, self-defeating and self-destructive behavior patterns are the product of faulty coping mechanisms.

In behavioral therapy, the patient assumes a new role. Together with the clinician, he searches for the various, especially ongoing, causes of his problems. He enters into a contract with his therapist on the goals which he wishes to realize and the manner in which they will attempt to achieve them. In contrast to psychoanalysis, the patient in behavioral therapy is often instructed to "try on" new behaviors like a set of new clothes. The application of these new behaviors to the actual circumstances of his own environment is encouraged as soon as possible. Proper therapeutic planning usually assures varying degrees of success, which increases the patient's self-confidence and optimism and motivates him to experiment with further new behaviors. This procedure subtly, but definitely, also aims at developing autonomy rather than chronic dependence upon the therapist.

Behavioral therapy for patients of this type offers a number of distinct advantages over classical psychoanalysis. First, it is uniquely suited for self-help in those individuals who consider some of their problems persistent and distressing, yet not serious enough to require professional psychiatric help. Currently, there are large numbers of well-written guidelines which the motivated reader can use alone, or with only minimal assistance, for favorably changing his own behavior or that of others.

Second, behavioral therapy uniquely offers the means of dealing directly with disorders of the autonomic nervous system. Indeed, the treatment of autonomic function through behavioral techniques has emerged as a separate discipline with its own specialists flying the flag of biofeedback.

Another advantage of behavioral therapy is that its language and its therapeutic measures are uncomplicated and correspond closely to common-sense thinking. Physicians who are "turned off" by Freudian methodology and terminology find the techniques easy to learn, readily applicable and very effective in clinical practice.

It is worth re-emphasizing that behavioral therapy stresses that problematic behavior is the product of one or more improper learning experiences and resultant faulty coping mechanisms. Recognition of the cause, unlearning the factors, and learning new coping mechanisms permits the individual to ultimately live in greater harmony with himself and others. Motivation to change behavior is essential along with the knowledge required to do so.

Despite its critics,[2–4] behavioral therapy has made important inroads at a time when we seek straightforward and cost-effective methods for helping large portions of our population who seek solutions to health problems without relinquishing their own involvement and sense of mastery and control over their own lives.

TECHNIQUES

The therapeutic rationale of behavioral therapy is based on the previously reviewed concepts. Since emotional and behavioral responses occur as conditioned reactions to certain stimulus situations, it is the goal of this therapy to substitute new, appropriate responses for the old, inappropriate ones. In ordinary learning, a new and desired behavior is combined sufficiently often with the stimulus situation so that, in time, the stimulus automatically evokes the new behavior, replacing the old, undesired behavior formerly conditioned to the same stimulus.

In behavioral therapy, the procedure is basically the same, with some variations. First, the old habit is unlearned by repeatedly practicing a more desirable behavior in response to the provocative stimulus. For example, a patient with angina pectoris is taught how to respond to his chest pain with a certain degree of thoughtful calmness instead of panic. Second, the patient is trained in relaxation techniques so that he will respond to certain known stressful situations with a reduction in muscle tone. Decreased muscle tone clearly inhibits emotional arousal centers in the brain. This facilitates the re-conditioning and modifying of emotional responses. Muscular relaxation is taught as a desired response to all emotionally distressing situations, since it reduces overreactive behavior. Overreactive behavior is taught as a totally inappropriate response, since it can only heat up the immediate environment and prevent optimal problem resolution. Third, as the patient's coping abilities increase, he is challenged with increasingly difficult stimulus situations. For example, if a patient developed angina when speaking up in a small group of individuals, he is brought to the point where he can deliver a lecture to a large audience and receive questions and criticism without pain.

The form of behavioral therapy just described is effective in a wide variety of anxiety or arousal responses. It is, however, predictably less effective in controlling global anxieties in persons with very weak or inadequate personalities. In these instances, broader therapeutic programs such as training in self-assertion may be required.

In accordance with the aforementioned concepts, behavior may also be determined by its consequences. A new, desired behavior will only be learned and maintained if the consequences it produces are positive and rewarding for the individual. In keeping with the adage that "nothing succeeds like success," the therapist structures the course of therapy in such a way as to provide the patient with rewarding experiences. One of the main techniques employed here is that of successive approximations of the desired behavior. For example, the patient with angina is helped to learn to speak to ever larger groups of people without experiencing pain. The role of the therapist is to motivate the patient to try on his new behaviors in his real life circumstances. Since the rewards for successful performance in the practical setting are far greater than in mere exercises in the therapist's office, reinforcement and motivation to extend the new behavior are correspondingly more powerful. Behavioral modification is best accomplished by reinforcing and rewarding good performance, rather than by punishing undesired behavior.

Modeling is an important agent for generating and maintaining behavior, and is perhaps best illustrated by childhood development. Children usually take after their parents; indeed, what a parent does is often more far-reaching in its consequences than what a parent says. The truth in this has long since been embodied in the saying, "One teaches best by example and less by words."

In the clinical area, consider the powerful nonverbal communication and instruction which a physician gives to a patient when he himself loses 40 pounds and stops smoking. By contrast, consider the credibility and influence of the overweight physician who, puffing away, lectures at length on the hazards of obesity and smoking.

The fourth concept of learning focuses on cognition. The term *cognition* denotes the process and content of thinking, i.e., ideas, opinions, beliefs, attitudes, preferences, wishes, expectations, interpretations, and evaluations. These forms of thinking take place as private or silent speech or "self-talk". The individual's self-talk mediates his perception of events and his ultimate response to them. It is what a person thinks (what he tells himself about what he perceives) that determines whether he has an appropriate or inappropriate autonomic, emotional, or behavioral response. It is this self-talk that determines whether he may be described as "thick-skinned" and resilient, or "thin-skinned" and overreactive to the same environmental happenings.

GOALS AND CRITERIA FOR OPTIMAL THOUGHT AND BEHAVIOR

One of the first objectives of the clinician is to discover the patient's self-talk and relate it to his problematic emotional responses and behavior. In speaking of the patient's reactions, he uses the terms *appropriate* and *inappropriate*, rather than *normal* and *abnormal*. The clinician must determine whether the patient's self-talk and its emotional and behavioral consequences are appropriate and serve the purpose of (1) perceiving and recognizing objective realities, including psycohlogical (among other things, are his expectations within reach? is it necessary that his expectations be met to the fullest extent possible?, can he get along satisfactorily if they are not met?); (2) protecting and maintaining health and life; (3) reaching long-term, as well as short-term, goals, such as success, inner harmony, and tranquility; (4) avoiding and terminating significant personal and emotional upsets and conflicts; and (5) avoiding and terminating significant conflicts with other people. Employing the above guidelines, one can determine whether individuals with emotional and behavioral problems harbor any inappropriate expectations and attitudes. For example, persons with inferiority feelings, depression and dependency behaviors usually tell themselves, "I must be thoroughly competent, adequate and achieving in all possible respects in order to consider myself worthy as a person," and "I need to be loved and approved of by every other person in my community." The individual who has resigned himself to being the way he is has the following self-talk: "My past is the all-important determinant of my present behavior. Because something once strongly affected my life, it must indefinitely continue to do so."

There are, however, even more fundamental self-talks which can have enormous counterproductive and self-destructive influences on people. One of these concerns a conception of the causes of emotional upset. How often does one hear "My boss makes me sick" or "Political trends frighten me" or "She is a pain in the neck"? This manner of thinking, which can be generalized as "People and events upset me," expresses a belief in a certain causal relationship between the perceived events and the emotional responses to them. Clearly, when an individual thinks this, he is ascribing to the event an inherent ability to directly and immediately determine his reactions. In some manner, the perception of this event (perhaps the behavior of another person) directly affects the activity in the autonomic nervous system and the function of those organs which it innervates.

This manner of thinking automatically results in very serious consequences. The individual, of necessity, externalizes his problems and detaches himself from any possible role in their origin. He thereby permanently conditions himself to become upset whenever and wherever the upsetting event occurs. Through his self-talk, he has programmed himself to react in a way much like a robot is conditioned to react when someone pushes its button.

Let us review an example of this manner of thinking in a typical post-infarction victim. A patient interrupted Dr. Witte in the middle of a stress management seminar and blurted out in tears:

"You can easily talk about stress and stress management! You're not in my shoes. I'm 48 years old and have just suffered a severe heart attack, which I would not have survived had not a doctor been close by when it happened. He tells me if I don't stop getting upset, I'll have another one which will finish me! But everything upsets me, especially work. The tensions, the deadlines, the incredible responsibilities which I have to shoulder — and my boss exploits me! All these things caused my heart attack. And the doctor says that I should avoid getting upset!

"He doesn't realize that I can't change my job; I'm too old and I need the money badly. I have two children to raise and a wife to support who couldn't cope without me! It is all so terrible and horrible; it's a real catastrophe!

"I know there are only two solutions to the problem. Hold out as long as I can and wait for my next and fatal heart attack or put a bullet through my head now!"

(This patient revealed later, in private talks, that he had already purchased a revolver and was caught up in an exhausting inner struggle not to use it.)

This case illustrates the self-destructive and paralyzing influences of self-talk which characterizes a legion of cardiac patients. Clearly, the patient views his heart attack and his stress as a direct consequence of the circumstances of his job. Since avoidance of the stressor is not possible and his self-talk provides him with only two equally unacceptable alternatives, it is quite predictable that this patient must live with a high level of anxiety, severe depression and a profound sense of hopelessness. Certainly, his fate could have been either a new infarct or suicide. Through his self-talk, the stage was set for a self-fulfilling prophecy.

It takes but a moment of reflection to realize that it is not the perceived event, but the manner in which we cope with it, that determines our emotional and behavioral responses. For one individual, a single insult may lead to a massive and perhaps fatal emotional arousal; in another, there may be mild irritation; in another, there may be cold indifference; and in yet another, there may be outright amusement. The lessons of life adequately demonstrate that there are emotionally "thin-skinned" and "thick-skinned" individuals. Some react to life's blows as a china doll would, while others respond as a rubber doll would.

By entering into therapy, the aforementioned patient was able to discard his own magical thinking. Happily, thus far he has averted either of his proposed tragic outcomes.

The course of his counseling was as follows. The patient was confronted with the belief that changes in his coping mechanisms were more likely possibilities than changes in his social environment. This was the initial and key focus in his stress management. Following a discussion of this, consideration was given to a number of his colleagues who worked in the same circumstances but had neither similar emotional reactions nor infarcts. The patient soon began to refer to himself as a thin-skinned person in terms of his reactions to his work situation as well as to other areas of his life. (The term *thin-skinned* is more acceptable to patients than *neurotic*.) He quickly recognized that he was externalizing his problems, blaming others for his stress, and that this was both illogical and self-defeating. He further recognized that getting greatly upset about failing to meet a deadline, for example, frequently hindered adjustment. The patient was then introduced to the reality that there is a gradation in intensity of negative emotional reactions with the aid of the list in Table I.

TABLE I

THIN-SKINNED REACTIONS	THICK-SKINNED REACTIONS
feelings of inferiority and worthlessness	dissatisfaction with single behaviors
overexcitedness; anxiety; panic	uneasiness; nervousness; concern
shock	painful awareness
rage; hate	anger; disliking
depression; suicidal mood	sadness; unhappiness
bitterness; cynicism	sadness; disappointment; frustration

Thin-skinned reactions impair the ability to deal con-structively with a given problem and may even create new ones. Thick-skinned reactions are still strong enough to motivate us toward seeking a solution, but do not impair successful resolution. This patient was then given assistance in becoming more thick-skinned in his reactions.

Following this first task of changing himself, he then explored with the therapist the possibilities of changing his environment. Not only did he learn that he was upsetting himself unduly over certain events, but he also learned that his own behavior was responsible for the continued exist-ence of those events. This was made apparent to the pa-tient in his passive acceptance of the demands of his boss (among them, to work overtime). It was not a question of being exploited, but of *permitting* himself to be exploited. As such, the focus was once again placed upon inadequate cop-ing behavior instead of on an environmental stressor. With further behavioral therapy, the patient became less emo-tionally overreactive and was able to eliminate some of his environmental stressors.

The goals of this form of therapy are twofold. The first

goal is to strengthen coping mechanisms in order to make the thin-skinned patient more resilient; the second is to eliminate or reduce the number and/or intensity of environmental stressors. The achievement of the first goal usually presents few problems for the motivated cardiac patient. The difficulty in realizing the second goal is then a function of the degree of control the therapist has over those environmental stressors in relationship to the patient. For example, adjustments in marital relationships are usually easier to facilitate than adjustments in the behavior of colleagues at work.

OTHER BEHAVIORAL TECHNIQUES

Transcendental Meditation

One of the more recent contemporary updates of older techniques is transcendental meditation (T.M.). T.M. is said to be easy to learn and requires no unusual physical or mental control, nor any dramatic changes in life-style. It requires 15 to 20 minutes twice daily, and is practiced in a comfortable seated position with eyes closed utilizing the systematic silent repetition of a mantra, or mystical word or sound. The latter effect has a tendency to temporarily detach the individual from his environment, producing a number of documented physiologic changes. These include decreased oxygen consumption, decreased CO_2 elimination, decreased minute ventilation and respiratory rate, while the respiratory quotient remains relatively constant.[5] When employed in the therapeutic sense, regular practice is reported to result in a significant reduction in blood pressure in borderline hypertensives (7 to 10 mm Hg).[6,7,8,9] The samples, however, have been small, and there is intersubject and intrasubject variation.[10] Few adverse side effects have been reported.[7]

The Relaxation Response

For many people, transcendental meditation is too "cultist", and is thus summarily rejected. As a non-cultist alternative, Benson and colleagues[11] have reported that similar physiologic responses can be induced by a similar technique employing the silent repetition of the number *one* as described below.

Eliciting the Relaxation Response

1. Sit quietly in a comfortable position.
2. Close the eyes.
3. Deeply relax all muscles.
4. Breathe in and out through the nose; repeat "one" silently.
5. Continue this for 10 to 20 minutes, once or twice daily.
6. When finished, sit quietly with the eyes closed and then gradually open them.
7. Maintain a passive attitude during the practice.

The technique has been described as producing a hypometabolic state which is different from pure sleep and represents the trophotropic response of Hess[12] observed in cats originally. The proposed mechanism for this response is (1) a decrease and counteraction in the flow of sympathetic nervous system activity, (2) integrated hypothalamic responses which tend to override sympathetic outflow, and (3) a possible increase in parasympathetic activity.[5] The physiologic effects are similar to those reported for transcendental meditation.

As a treatment mode, it may have value in selected cases where excessive sympathetic nervous system activity is observed by the physician. In hypertension, for example, there may be a significant decrease in systolic and diastolic pressures, even when individuals are on antihypertensive agents.[13] There are no known untoward effects of utilizing this technique in the presence of antihypertensive agents. One should, however, be warned of the risk of using ganglionic or beta blockade. Such potent antihypertensive agents that impede sympathetic activity or function in a manner similar to blocked sympathetic activity might be dangerous to the individual who can significantly decrease sympathetic activity through relaxation techniques.

Additionally, this technique has found some use in ventricular ectopic activity. Several investigators have reported a reduction in the frequency of premature ventricular beats in pilot studies.[14,15] There are also individual case reports in which the technique appeared to be an important adjunct to the management of potentially terminal ventricular arrhythmias.[16]

It will also be recalled that in the physiology of stress, the importance of the sympathetic nervous system was reviewed with regard to the multiple pathways, innervations and effects involving the heart. Therefore, there appears to be room for continuing investigation with regard to the use of similar techniques in effectively reducing hyperactive sympathetic flow. When cost is a factor, the technique can be simply applied as outlined above.

Progressive Relaxation is another non-pharmacologic approach by which one induces a low level of muscle tone in major muscle groups by learning discriminative control of skeletal muscles. The technique was developed and popularized by Jacobson[17] in the 1930s. Recently, investigators have employed it as an antihypertensive behavior modification technique with some success in what must again be considered pilot studies.[18-20]

Biofeedback

"Biofeedback is the use of modern instrumentation to give a person better moment-to-moment information about a specific physiologic process that is under the control of the

central nervous system but not clearly or accurately perceived. In the terminology of servo systems, such information has been called feedback. Such information about a
biologic process is called biofeedback".[21] It has been demonstrated that individuals can be trained to regulate such
functions as heart rate, blood pressure, cardiac output,
blood flow to skeletal muscle, skin temperatures, sweat
gland activity, gastric and intestinal processes and so
forth.[22,23]

The mechanisms of action remain to be clarified at this
time. The physiologic action implies that almost any
physiologic function can be changed through conscious
processes. Few, if any, side effects have been reported for
hypertensive patients, but one cannot overlook the importance of agents that block sympathetic nervous outflow at
any level, or that parallel such activity in antihypertensive
therapy. Its use indicates caution when any biofeedback
technique is employed.

Biofeedback is a tool which has potential for elucidat-
ing mechanisms as well as for therapy. However, research
has only begun to scratch the surface of this potential. As
our instrumentation, particularly noninvasive monitoring
of physiologic functioning, becomes more sophisticated,
the theory and techniques of biofeedback will provide
the guidelines for innovative research into mind-body
relationships.

Group Therapy

Group therapy offers a number of decided advantages
over individual therapy in that it permits more efficient use
of the therapist's time and skills. In individual therapy, the
clinician observes the patient's behavior in an admittedly
artificial situation. Placing the patient into a group forces
him into social interaction, which is a good means of gaining
critical in situ information on the nature and extent of his
interpersonal conflicts and the means by which he copes

with them. In group therapy, the individual is no longer simply a patient, but is also a therapist. In witnessing other people's problems and their struggles in dealing with them, and by offering empathy, insight and practical assistance to them, he is given growth experiences which cannot be approached in individual therapy. Furthermore, he receives feedback and help from his peers, which may often be a more potent influence in changing his behavior than interaction with the therapist alone.

These realities form the basis of our conviction that a program of comprehensive, preventive and rehabilitative cardiology must offer the patient (who is suited for such an experience) the opportunity for participation in group interaction. Ideally, both individual and group therapy would be the best approach.

Improperly conducted group experiences can be shattering to a person; not only emotional scarring, but also psychotic breaks and suicides, have occurred in encounter groups run by inadequately trained leaders, for example. Therefore, the physician utilizing group therapy must have considerable knowledge of, and confidence in, the qualifications and competence of the therapist to whom he delegates his authority.

Hypnosis

Hypnosis has not been demonstrated to be a proven adjunct or therapeutic technique in behavioral modification. Although there have been some impressive short-term results in the studies done on smoking cessation, maintenance of this behavior has been a problem.[24,25]

Others

Some of the more mundane but useful forms of behavior modification include adjustments which improve the quality of life. Among these are such things as lunch away from work with individuals who come from other businesses or professions and who agree to discuss non-work topics. Another is performing one function at a time and limiting polyphasic activity. A third is to plan some idleness during each day. A fourth is to take time for activities that are entirely self-serving and personally rewarding. The latter may involve a range of activities from reading to crafts of various types, exercise, participation in community programs, taking time for humor, and planning by the calendar rather than the stop watch. It is often useful for the heavily scheduled individual to schedule some time for absolutely nothing. The latter can be greatly assisted by one's secretarial staff and referred to as "an important conference," "an emergency call," "out of the office," or, for even longer periods, "out of town." This gives the person time to stop, take time out and return with a better plan and proper priorities. This allows one to plan one's life rather than to react to it.

Frequently, the major problem in achieving any of the aforementioned goals is the alleviation of feelings of guilt. The latter develops on the basis of the Calvinistic concern of most productive people. They often feel they must constantly be doing something or they aren't being productive or useful. The physician's counsel in alleviating such guilt is the first step in modifying behavior. This can often be aided by pointing out how non-human, mechanical, robot-like behavior is self-destructive. Therefore, one should not feel guilty about trying to preserve oneself as a human being by employing human rewards.

REFERENCES

1. Puzzling out man's ascent. *Time* **110**:64-67, 1977.
2. Carkhuff, R., and Berenson, B.: *Beyond Counseling and Therapy.* New York: Holt, Rinehart and Winston, 1967.
3. Koestler, A.: *The Ghost in the Machine.* New York: Macmillan Co., 1967.

4. Breger, L., and McGaugh, J.L.: Critique and reformulation of "learning theory" approaches to psychotherapy and neuroses. *Psychological Bulletin* **63**:338-358, 1965.

5. Beary, J.F., Benson, H., and Klemchuk, H.P.: A simple psychophysiologic technique which elicits the hypometabolic changes of the relaxation response. *Psychosomatic Med.* **36**:115-120, 1974.

6. Benson, H., and Wallace, R.K.: Decreased blood pressure in hypertensive subjects who practice meditation. *Circulation* **46**: Supplement II: 130, 1972.

7. Benson, H., Rosner, B.A., Marzetta, B.R., et al: Decreased blood pressure in borderline hypertensive patients who practice meditation. *J. Chronic Dis.* **27**:163-169, 1974.

8. Benson, H., Marzetta, B.R., and Rosner, B.A.: Decreased blood pressure associated with the regular elicitation of the relaxation response: A study of hypertensive subjects. In R.S. Eliot (Ed.): *Stress and the Heart.* Mt. Kisco, New York: Futura Publishing Co., 1974, pp. 293-302.

9. Blackwell, B., Bloomfield, S., Gartside, P., et al: Transcendental meditation in hypertension. *Lancet* **1**:223-226, 1976.

10. Shapiro, A.P., Schwartz, G.E., Ferguson, D.C.E., et al: Behavioral methods in the treatment of hypertension. A review of their clinical status. *Ann. Intern. Med.* **86**:626-636, 1977.

11. Benson, H.: *The Relaxation Response.* New York: William Morrow and Co., 1975.

12. Hess, W.R.: *Functional Organization of the Diencephalon.* New York: Grune and Stratton, 1957.

13. Benson, H., Rosner, B.A., Marzetta, B.R., and Klemchuk, H.M.: Decreased blood pressure in pharmacologically treated hypertensive patients who regularly elicited the relaxation response. *Lancet* **1**:289-291, 1974.

14. Benson, H., Alexander, S., and Feldman, C.L.: Decreased premature ventricular contractions through use of the relaxation response in patients with stable ischaemic heart disease. *Lancet* **1**:380, 1975.

15. Lown, B., Verrier, R.L., and Rabinowitz, S.H.: Neural and psychologic mechanisms and the problem of sudden cardiac death. *Amer. J. Cardiol.* **39**:890-902, 1977.

16. Lown, B., Temte, J.V., Reich, P., et al: Basis for recurring ventricular fibrillation in the absence of coronary heart disease and its management. *New Eng. J. Med.* **294**:623-629, 1976.

17. Jacobson, E.: *Progressive Relaxation.* Chicago: University of Chicago Press, 1938.

18. Dearbler, H.L.: Fidel, E., Dillenkoffer, R.L.: The use of relaxation and hypnosis in lowering high blood pressure: *Amer. J. Clinical Hypnosis* **16**:75-83, 1973.

19. Shoemaker, J.E., and Tsato, D.L.: The effects of muscle relaxation of blood pressure of essential hypertensives. *Behavior Research Therapy* **13**:29-43, 1975.

20. Redmond, D.P., Gaylor, M.S., McDonald, R.H., et al: Blood pressure and heart rate response to verbal instructions and relaxation in hypertension. *Psychosomatic Med.* **36**:285-297, 1974.

21. Miller, N.E.: Biofeedback: Evaluation of a new technique. *New Eng. J. Med.* **290**:684-685, 1974.

22. Blanchard, E.B., Young, L.D., and Haynes, M.R.: A simple feedback system for the treatment of elevated blood pressure. *Behavior Therapy* **6**:241-245, 1975.

23. Shapiro, D., and Schwartz, G.E.: Biofeedback and visceral learning: Clinical applications. *Seminars in Psychiatry* **4**:171-184, 1972.

24. Sanders, S.: Mutual group hypnosis and smoking. *Amer. J. Clinical Hypnosis* **20**:131-135, 1977.

25. Shewchuk, L.A., Dubren, R., Burton, D., et al: Preliminary observations on an intervention program for heavy smokers. *International Journal of the Addictions* **12**:323-336, 1977.

CHAPTER 6

PHARMACOLOGIC THERAPY

Both anxiety and depression are frequent components or precursors of coronary disease. In certain instances of anxiety or depression it may be desirable to temporarily employ psychotropic agents that blunt the afferent or efferent portion of the stress loop or both. Reduction of anxiety or depression may be required to liberate sufficient intellectual reserve for more constructive purposes. A variety of agents are available that fulfill, to varying degrees, the aforementioned goals. Before using these agents, however, one must balance the potential side effects and risks with the expected benefits.

ANTI-ANXIETY AGENTS

The coronary patient often demonstrates profound signs and symptoms of anxiety. Cardiovascular indicators such as palpitations, tachyarrhythmias, precordial pain or syncope are among those well known to the clinician. Anxiety may be either overt or covert, and, in the latter, the patient may not communicate feelings of anxiety. Indeed, in a harried clinical atmosphere, covert anxiety may be totally masked with the exception of its cardiovascular manifestations.

Usually the physician will recognize anxiety by observation during the history input. Indicators of anxiety include restlessness, hyperventilation, tense and worried faces, excessive perspiration or, in many instances, information from a third party (often the spouse). The physician can

107

also rely to a certain degree on his own sense of discomfort. The mere presence of an anxious individual can create similar reactions in the physician, thereby alerting him to the patient's problem.

In the setting of the coronary care unit, we may assume that all patients are anxious, especially within the first 24 hours of the acute event. Therefore, they must be treated accordingly. It is usually advantageous to prescribe tranquilizers in such patients. It may be desirable to keep them drowsy, and, for this reason, the medicines should be given regularly and not on demand. Chlordiazepoxide or diazepam appear to be the most useful agents in my experience. I prefer the latter because it does not mimic the effects of catecholamines. At bedtime, it is appropriate to double the dose. As a substitute for diazepam, flurazepam may be utilized for two or three nights following the acute infarction. Thereafter, it may interfere with sleep and contribute to the psychoneurotic reactions that are frequent within intensive care settings. While attempts to utilize hypnosis have been generally ineffective, autorelaxation techniques such as meditation may be helpful, but in this setting should be viewed as adjuncts rather than major therapeutic avenues.

Among the commonly used tranquilizing agents are chlordiazepoxide and diazepam, which are both considered safe and effective. Flurazepam appears less safe and less effective and, therefore, I limit its use to two or three nights post-infarction. The mechanism of action of these agents is to reduce anxiety by selectively depressing the limbic system activity. They induce muscle relaxation by depressing polysynaptic reflex pathways. They also have anticonvulsant properties. Their effectiveness is enhanced by the rapidity with which they are absorbed from all routes.

Diazepam decreases urinary adrenal excretion following acute myocardial infarction.[1] In addition, it has some beneficial hemodynamic side effects for the cardiovascular patient. It has a nitroglycerin-like action, which, the reader will recall, is dominantly a medical tourniquet function.[2] Its pharmacology includes venodilatation and pooling, thereby decreasing left ventricular filling pressure (preload). These results are accompanied by decreases in left ventricular end diastolic pressure, aortic pressure, myocardial wall tension, and the tension time index. There is no change in heart rate and, therefore, the use of this agent results in decreased myocardial oxygen consumption (MVO_2). Its side effects are relatively few, with the exception of interference with REM activity after prolonged periods of use, but toxic effects usually require much higher than ordinary clinical doses. The patient receiving diazepam must be cautioned about activities requiring complete mental alertness. Concomitant ingestion of alcohol is contraindicated. It must also be remembered that older patients may show a reduced tolerance to diazepam.

The well-known correlation between plasma and urinary concentration of catecholamines makes it probable that using diazepam to treat patients with acute myocardial infarction causes a decreased plasma level of catecholamines.[1] This may be of considerable importance because increased plasma levels of catecholamines are frequently seen during acute myocardial infarction and are known to induce ventricular arrhythmias and contribute to cardiogenic shock.[1] Vetter and colleagues[3] have also demonstrated elevated concentrations of free fatty acids and cortisol during the time of acute myocardial infarction. Persistent elevation of free fatty acids increases myocardial oxygen demands (MVO_2) and predisposes to ventricular arrhythmias.[4,5]

Barbiturates have been utilized for many decades. Among these, phenobarbital has been among the most frequently used. It has a cumulative effect and a tendency to dull the mentation. It is excreted dominantly by the kidney and, therefore, is reasonably dependent upon adequate renal output. Varying dosage intervals are required depending upon the agent employed (pentobarbital, amobarbital, secobarbital). Frequently, the withdrawal of these agents is followed by headaches and depression, as well as other side effects. It is important to keep in mind that barbiturates interfere with the plasma half-life of coumarin, and for this reason may be contraindicated in those circumstances where coumarin is employed.[6]

Substituted phenothiazines are often of use where heavy tranquilization is required. Among those available, I prefer chlorpromazine in this setting. Although there is a very slight hypotensive effect, it is not a major risk when the patient is at bed rest. On beginning ambulation, however, orthostatic hypotension frequently accompanies rehabilitation of cardiac victims or any patient at chronic bed rest. Since orthostasis is a side effect of such agents, caution is advised in this setting.

As a general rule, PRN orders are rarely adequate for any antianxietal agents. Organizing therapy in this fashion may create anxiety in itself.

ANTI-DEPRESSANT AGENTS

It is well recognized that overt depression follows acute myocardial infarction and is self-limited in most instances. It usually begins on the second day of infarction following the realization that survival is a very good possibility.[7] The dynamics of such a depression involve a constellation of individual and collective concerns experienced by the patient. Among these are the loss of autonomy, inability to control the environment, emasculation, fear of invalidism, and the fear of loss of income. Recognizing that depression of this variety is usually limited, one of the most important means of management is positive reinforcement in words and in optimism by the physician and his staff. Depression is also a frequent event following open-heart procedures or in hospitalizations for cardiovascular illnesses which are of a prolonged nature. Obviously, it may be seen in outpatient settings as well, and is a frequent covert precursor of initial or recurrent infarction or sudden death.

The relief of symptoms of depression is far from prompt. Indeed, it may take from three to ten days or up to three weeks to achieve adequate therapeutic management by pharmacologic methods. In myocardial infarction, depression may continue for as long as six months to a year and a half, depending upon many individual and environmental factors. When protracted, psychiatric consultation may be of value.

The mechanism of action of tricyclic anti-depressants in human beings is not known. Monoamine oxidase (MAO) inhibitors produce a euphoric stimulation and an increase in the norepinephrine pool within the brain. The cardiovascular side effects are tachycardia, palpitations, arrhythmias, orthostatic hypotension, ankle edema, bizarre electrocardiographic changes, syncope and even the precipitation of congestive heart failure.

MAO inhibitors can be used, however, in hypertension, in direct blockade of sympathetic ganglia, and in angina pectoris in coronary dilation, if the latter is ever demonstrated to be of physiologic significance in the relief of myocardial ischemia. These agents do have many unfortunate drug and food interactions which limit their effectiveness and usage.

BETA BLOCKING AGENTS

For the individual with bonafide evidence of ischemic heart disease or essential hypertension and no contraindications, it may be necessary to blunt the effect of excessive stressful input in order to avoid or diminish the state of chronic visceral-vascular readiness. One of the major advances over the past decade has been the selective utilization of beta blocking agents in the control of angina and mild hypertension. In the former, many national and international studies have been conducted which demonstrate their efficacy in the relief of pain primarily by the control and reduction of myocardial oxygen consumption (MVO_2). The effectiveness of beta blockade for two such apparently different disease states has always intrigued me with regard to the influence of stress in these apparently divergent pathophysiologic states.

In several foreign countries, beta blocking agents have been satisfactorily employed and investigated for over a decade in the management of essential hypertension. Approval for their use in the United States has been limited to arrhythmias, idiopathic hypertrophic subaortic stenosis, pheochromocytoma and angina pectoris. Only recently have they been approved for the treatment of hypertension.

The mode of action of these agents remains imperfectly defined. Yet it can be said that there is a vascular component of action which is suggested by their effect on the blood pressure in the reduction of total peripheral resistance.[8] The long-term adaptation of the peripheral resistance to the diminished cardiac output appears to be suitably blocked. The result is that, following a period of diminished cardiac output, the compensatory increase in peripheral resistance is abolished by these agents.[9] Their effectiveness in decreasing blood pressure correlates well with the pre-existing plasma renin activity and with the degree of renin suppression produced by the agents.[10]

Beta blocking agents also demonstrate a powerful central nervous system effect which, although it does not "tranquilize" the individual, reduces the transmission of external stressful stimuli through the efferent arc of the sympathetic nervous system. They are well known to produce sinus bradycardia, a decrease in the rate of development of tension of the left ventricle, and to produce a mild coronary vasoconstriction which is more than compensated for by the former pharmacologic effects.

In the end, what is accomplished is a blunting of the

state of visceral-vascular readiness, or the so-called alarm reaction. The effectiveness of this blunting from the standpoint of the patient's perception is often interesting. Frequently, an individual who has a high state of alertness, aggressiveness or arousal will return to the physician and inquire, "Was I placed on a tranquilizer?" Such a phenomenon is of frequent therapeutic use to the physician, for it may indicate clearly the state of alarm and visceral-vascular readiness not only to the physician but also to the patient. When the patient realizes that the normal state of arousal is that which is accomplished in him only by reasonable beta blockade, the stage may be set for behavior modification. In such cases, the beta blocking agent acts as a pharmacologic "two-by-four" to give insight and to draw the patient's attention to his problem. The goal of tranquility is often adequate motivation toward the self-control of the chronic state of visceral-vascular readiness. I have often used this pharmacologic "two-by-four" as a "preview of coming attractions." Used in this manner, it adds to the motivational thrust.

Beta blockers are known to be contraindicated in chronic bradycardias, AV conduction defects or where myocardial contractility is reduced. In the former two, this is a result of the negative chronotropic effects of propranolol, and in the latter, its negative inotropic effects. Furthermore, the resultant diminished cardiac output may aggravate peripheral arterial insufficiency. Finally, beta blocking agents may be contraindicated in certain respiratory conditions, such as asthma and upper respiratory infections (the common cold), because they inhibit the beta receptors in the bronchial smooth muscle.

One of the most important cautions with beta blockade involves the care with which it should be withdrawn from therapy. It is now well established that acute myocardial infarction and sudden death can be engendered by the sudden withdrawal of beta blockade.[11] The release of its inhibiting effect may bring about a rebound of heart rate, inotropism, and enhanced peripheral resistance, all of which can dramatically increase MVO_2. In addition, the rapid rebound in peripheral resistance may be reflected in an acute hypertensive state. Complications such as acute myocardial infarction, sudden death or cerebral vascular accident are indeed an unfortunate result of overlooking these important considerations.

Many new beta blocking agents, which have differing actions and side effects than propranolol, are receiving approval for clinical trials. Some of these will find approval by the Food and Drug Administration and will become available in clinical practice. In the near future, the physician should have a variety of therapeutic options when prescribing a beta blocking agent.

As described in the above paragraphs, tranquilization and beta blockade are used in a highly selective, and usually temporary, fashion. When psychoneurosis, psychosis, or chronic dependency appears likely, the matter has gone beyond temporary supportive measures and into psychotherapeutic management. In the latter instance (less than five percent of cases), psychiatric consultation can be of great value.

USE OF ALCOHOL

Today alcohol is frequently utilized as a tranquilizer or relaxing agent. Unfortunately, it is frequently overutilized and abused in this regard. Acute alcoholism may be accompanied by the release of free fatty acids, catecholamines, depression of myocardial contractility and elevation of myocardial enzymes (transaminase CPK MB), thereby indicating its potential to induce necrosis. As mentioned earlier, elevation of free fatty acids may induce an increase in myocardial oxygen requirements (MVO_2) and may even induce ventricular arrhythmias.[1,4,5] For the patient with coronary heart disease or hypertension, alcohol usage should be a major clinical consideration. In addition, the caloric contribution of alcohol and its substitution for food may support and sustain obesity as well as chronic hyper-triglyceridemia. Thus, "alcoholic" tranquilization is accomplished at the expense of untoward biochemical and hemodynamic derangement with excessive caloric intake. Furthermore, the effect is more akin to pithing than tranquilizing.

A more ideal agent would be one which produces tranquilization and relaxation with a diminished biochemical, hemodynamic and caloric impact. Such an agent is common dry table wine. The ethanol content per ounce is approximately one-third that of hard liquor, and six ounces contain approximately 140 calories (based on 12 percent alcohol content). When sipped and not "slurped", the blood alcohol level is gradually elevated, the tongue is loosened and communication is generally enhanced. The let-down is gradual. The individual becomes relaxed rather than "chemically pithed", which is a result of one or two martinis (not to mention the 250 calories per drink). Ten to twelve ounces of dry white or red wine provides a caloric intake of approximately 230 to 275 calories and an alcohol content equivalent to three to four ounces of hard liquor. A five-ounce glass of wine (115 calories) can add a pleasing touch to a weight reduction diet. Thus, in the hospital, I suggest that the patient begin to replace hard liquor with five to six ounces of dry table wine (white or red). This intake may be increased, but should not exceed 12 ounces per day on release from the hospital. The level of acceptance by patients has been extremely high, and is usually accompanied by the elimination of hard liquor from the diet and greater facility in control of weight.

One may ask why beer could not be considered equal to wine in this capacity. First, the alcohol concentration is such (5 to 6 percent) that an excessive number of calories must be consumed to produce the desirable relaxing effect. Beer contains approximately 210 calories per 12 ounces. Its relatively high carbohydrate content has a tendency to rapidly raise blood glucose and, on withdrawal, induces a reactive hypoglycemia accompanied by an increased appetite. It is possible that some of the new so-called "light" or low calorie beers may alter its usefulness in this respect.

Obviously, any form of management requires a knowledge of the individual's taste and preferences. For those who prefer beer to wine, the light beers may become a valid option and are worth a therapeutic try. The availability of reasonably good, low cost domestic wines has brought them into a reasonably good posture with the brewer's art on a competitive price basis. The utilization of wine during the social hour and at the dinner table has been gratifying. It helps achieve the goals of improved communication, weight control and so forth.

REFERENCES

1. Melsom, M., Andreassen, P., Melsom, H., et al: Diazepam in acute myocardial infarction. Clinical effects and effects on catecholamines, free fatty acids, and cortisol. *Brit. Heart J.* **38**:804-810, 1976.

2. Ikram, H., Rubin, A.P., and Jewkes, R.F.: Effects of diazepam on myocardial blood flow of patients with and without coronary artery disease. *Brit. Heart J.* **35**:626, 1973.

3. Vetter, N.J., Strange, R.C., Adams, W., and Oliver, M.F.: Initial metabolic and hormonal response to acute myocardial infarction. *Lancet* **1**:284, 1974.

4. Oliver, M.F., Kurien, V.A., and Greenwood, T.W.: Relation between serum-free-fatty-acids and arrhythmias and death after acute myocardial infarction. *Lancet* **1**:710, 1968.

5. Rutenberg, H.L., Pamintuan, J.C., and Soloff, L.A.: Serum-free-fatty-acids and their relation to complications after acute myocardial infarction. *Lancet* **2**:559, 1969.

6. Hunninghake, D.B., and Azarnoff, D.L.: Drug interactions with warfarin. *Arch. Intern. Med.* **121**:349, 1968.

7. Cassem, N.H., and Hackett, T.P.: Psychiatric consultation in a coronary care unit. *Ann. Intern. Med.* **75**:9-14, 1971.

8. Frohlich, E.D., Tarazi, R.C., Dustan, H.P., and Page, I.H.: The paradox of beta-adrenergic blockade in hypertension. *Circulation* **37**:417-423, 1968.

9. Tarazi, R.C., and Dustan, H.P.: Beta-adrenergic blockade in hypertension: Practical and theoretical implications of long-term hemodynamic variations. *Amer. J. Cardiol.* **29**:633-640, 1972.

10. Buhler, F.R., Laragh, J.H., Baer, L., et al: Propranolol inhibition of renin secretion: A specific approach to diagnosis and treatment of renin-dependent hypertensive diseases. *New Eng. J. Med.* **287**:1209-1214, 1972.

11. Alderman, E.L., Coltart, D.J., Wettach, G.E., and Harrison, D.C.: Coronary artery syndromes after sudden propranolol withdrawal. *Ann. Intern. Med.* **81**:625-627, 1974.

CHAPTER 7

EXERCISE

At the outset, it is important to indicate that within the practice of medicine, enthusiasm for exercise ranges from religious fervor to apathy to hostile opposition. Naturally, when such a variety of opinions are articulated by a chorus of silver-tongued and variously muscled orators, the truth must lie somewhere between the alpha and omega. Indeed, sound facts are extremely difficult to sift out of the near cultist enthusiasm which has, in some instances, proclaimed appropriate exercise to be a cure for everything from constipation to coronary atherosclerosis. It is, therefore, important to define what exercise is and what its potential therapeutic value may be; and furthermore, to indicate that, as with any therapeutic agent, exercise has some important benefits but at the same time some limiting, toxic or even fatal side effects.

Within the scope of this text we are concerned primarily with patients who have ischemic or infarcted hearts and/or who are hypertensive. It is well known that these individuals usually have diseased coronary vessels and, in certain instances, damaged left ventricles as well. In other instances, there may be hypertrophy of the left ventricle. Obviously, such individuals have limited exercise capabilities. It is equally important to recognize that the asymptomatic "worried well" person will often require similar evaluation and can be considered along with those discussed in this chapter.

119

GOALS

The first question, then, to be asked is, what are the goals to be accomplished by an exercise program for any of the aforementioned patient groups? The first goal should be to condition the cardiovascular system, thereby permitting the individual to perform external work at a lower myocardial oxygen cost. The second goal would be to blunt, ameliorate or suppress the chronic state of visceral-vascular readiness which is a part of the alarm reaction. The third would be to improve the self confidence and "joie de vivre" of the indivdual — a phenomenon which, although subjective, anecdotal, and elusive, is universally reported.

OTHER PHYSIOLOGIC CHANGES

Some of the additional fringe benefits involve the peripheral vascular system and the oxygen transport system. There is often a decrease in the peripheral arterial resistance in the labile phase of early hypertension.[1] The second fringe benefit is an improvement in the peripheral oxygen transport system involving the red cells and the skeletal muscles. In the former, there is an increase in 2,3-diphosphoglyceric acid within the red cell.[2] This substance is known to enhance the facility with which oxygen is released by hemoglobin. In the latter, there is an increase in the concentration of skeletal muscle myoglobin, thereby facilitating oxygen transport at the skeletal muscle level.[3] The end result is enhanced oxygen release and reception, and, therefore, enhanced efficiency of the oxygen transport system. It remains unknown whether there is an increase in the quantity of myocardial myoglobin in man with exercise. There appears to be considerable evidence for this in animals.[4]

SOME PREVALENT MYTHS

Several myths have dominated the field of exercise that need to be dispelled. These include the myth that coronary arteries dilate as the result of exercise, thereby increasing coronary flow potential. Clarence Demar, the marathon runner, is the classic argument for the protagonists; the counter argument is that of Paavo Nurmi, three time Olympic marathon winner, who was ravaged with atherosclerosis in his late fifties.

A second myth to be dispelled is that exercise produces enhanced collateral circulation in the myocardium. Experimental and clinical evidence clearly demonstrates that collateral circulation develops under two distinct circumstances. In the first, there is an obstruction to flow based on coronary stenosis creating a high pressure source and a low pressure sink.[5] This gradual process is accompanied by the opening of inherent collaterals which lie fallow until pressure gradients call them into action. The second major mechanism is chronic hypoxia.[5] In this setting, hypoxia for 24 hours per day is required. The two common situations where this can be found are in residents living 7,000 feet above sea level or in chronic anemias. The opening of collateral circulation requires approximately 36 hours in animals.[6] It is assumed that this figure would be the same for man. Intermittent exercise, albeit strenuous and of several hours duration, is not sufficient to induce collateral circulation by hypoxia. These observations are supported predominantly by studies in animals, but also by autopsy studies in man.[7-9] Thus, the only two known common denominators for the development of collaterals include significant chronic coronary stenosis and/or hypoxia.

AEROBIC VERSUS ISOMETRIC EXERCISE

One of the first requirements in preparing an exercise prescription is a firm understanding of the major physiologic forms of exercise, aerobic and isometric. Aerobic exercise is accomplished by moving the body through space employing primarily the large muscle groups. This form of exercise includes walking, bicycle riding, swimming and jogging, for example. Isometric exercise is accomplished by moving muscle groups against each other or in a weight-lifting manner. Metaphorically, aerobic exercise is like driving one's automobile in overdrive within the 55 mph speed limit; isometric exercise is comparable to speeding with the brakes fully applied.

Normal aerobic exercise is accompanied by a reduction in the peripheral resistance and a sizeable increase in cardiac output and oxygen consumption.[10] This is brought about primarily by an increase in the heart rate and enhanced oxygen extraction associated with a reduction in peripheral resistance. In more highly conditioned individuals, there may be a slight to moderate increase in the stroke volume as well.[11] In addition, there is decreased blood flow to the viscera and nonworking muscle groups, and with further conditioning, there is an improvement of oxygen uptake capability.[10]

By contrast, isometric exercise or sustained muscle contraction, such as weight lifting with little or no motion, results in cardiovascular reflexes and hemodynamic responses that differ dramatically from those associated with aerobic exercise. Initiation of such muscular activity is accompanied by withdrawal of vagal tone and, within seconds, there is a tachycardia and an acute hypertensive response.[12] This reflex is powerful in that it can override normally set baroreceptors. A sudden increase in myocardial wall tension is accompanied by increased peripheral resistance (afterload), which combines to markedly increase myocardial oxygen demands disproportionate to the modest increase in cardiac output. An additional concern in hypertensive patients is their overresponsiveness to isometric exercise when compared to normotensives.[13] This hyperresponsiveness carries risks not only in myocardial oxygenation, but also in the rapid development of tension in the arterial wall which increases the risk of an intimal break or rupture. Another disadvantage of isometric exercise is that it generally taxes myocardial metabolism without facilitating oxygen delivery or training the cardiovascular system. Thus, isometric exercise markedly limits the duration of such activity before compromising myocardial integrity. Isometrics have also been shown to be highly arrhythmiagenic in people with heart disease, perhaps from reflex catecholamine release, and, therefore, are usually prohibited in any cardiovascular conditioning program.[14]

PHYSIOLOGIC UNCOUPLING

One of the major adjuncts of exercise is the relief of emotional stress.[10] For the purpose of this discussion, let us reiterate that stress is defined as an obviously painful or adverse force which may induce distress or strain upon both the emotional and physical makeup.[15] The resolution of this adverse force cannot be met by traditional fight or flight responses owing to societal or behavioral constraints. When unresolved, this results in a constant state of visceral-vascular readiness (the chronic alarm reaction). The outcome of this state depends upon the ability of the individual to adapt in a constructive or self-destructive fashion. In the former, health would be anticipated to prevail; in the latter, various disease states, frequently involving the cardiovascular system, may be provoked or enhanced.

Man typically responds to a stressful stimulus by first mobilizing the cardiovascular system to meet the anticipated metabolic needs. Next, there is an engagement of the musculoskeletal system to resolve the "fight or flight" dilemma. In essence, where survival or physical protection is the root of the stressful stimulus, the hypothalamic defense reactions are admirably suited to sustain the general well-being of the individual. However, in the case of most twentieth century stress, a successful resolution of the alarm reaction is needed, not so much to insure physical survival, but more so to facilitate psychosocial adjustment. In contemporary circumstances, resolution of the stress response by musculoskeletal involvement (fight or flight) is not usually a socially acceptable option. In this setting, the mobilized cardiovascular system is dissociated from the effector organs in the response mechanism, the musculoskeletal system. Neurogenically mediated changes in blood chemistry and myocardial metabolism are thus prolonged, and the cardiovascular system is maintained in extended, unresolved and potentially harmful periods of readiness. In the absence of augmented vasodilatation subsequent to muscular exercise, the state of cardiovascular preparedness is not discharged. The heart and vascular system are thus subjected to workloads far in excess of that expected during aerobic muscular activity. Prolonged, unresolved stress with dissociated cardiovascular and muscular systems eventuates in prolonged cardiovascular strain.

To be more specific, the stress adaptation process is comprised of three parts: (1) the stimulus or stress provocation; (2) the integrating process of the CNS; and (3) the effector response mechanism of the organism. When examining the pathologic consequences of chronic cardiac stress, it is toward the latter two components that attention will be directed.

Stress situations influence, and are influenced by, the higher centers of the central nervous system, and cardiac responses are mediated through neuronal and hormonal mechanisms. Neuronal channels include the vagal and sympathetic systems. The hormonal mechanisms involve both the adrenal and pituitary glands, and are responsible for one of the earliest physiological responses to stress, energy substrate mobilization. During the initial response to stress, adrenal medullary catecholamines activate glucose and fat stores. Pituitary hormones such as ACTH activate adrenal cortical release of glucocorticoids, which enhance substrate availability and tissue metabolism. Conservation of salt and water is also promoted by adrenal and pituitary secretions of aldosterone and ADH respectively.

During the stress adaptation process, neuroendocrine mediators cause significant alterations in circulatory dynamics. This increases selective vasodilatation, blood pressure, cardiac output, heart rate and myocardial contractility while it diminishes myocardial potassium. It must be noted that the aforementioned hemodynamic effects are based largely on experimental data. Chronic hypothalamic stimulation in animal experiments inhibits autoregulation of vasodilatation resulting in increased skeletal muscle blood flow and cardiac output with elevated blood pressure.[16] Blood flow is not only increased under sympathetic control, but is selectively redistributed as well. Preferential vasodilatation occurs in skeletal muscle with compensatory decreases in splanchnic and renal flow. By contrast, cerebral blood flow and oxygen uptake are unaffected by stress-induced circulatory redistribution.[17]

The chronic cardiovascular readiness state also appears to predispose to hypertension. Acute stress-induced elevations in aortic pressure are governed by homeometric autoregulatory processes in which increased developed myocardial contractility is not associated with corresponding alterations in left ventricular size and end diastolic volume.[18] Increased ventricular contractility, in turn, significantly decreases myocardial potassium concentration. Stress-induced homeometric autoregulation, therefore, may predispose to cardiac rhythm disorders via disturbances of myocardial electrolyte balance.

One of the most common and pronounced alterations in myocardial performance during the stress response is tachycardia. Increased frequency of contraction is regulated by sympathetic stimulation and will be accompanied by a release of myocardial catecholamines.[19] The potential for rhythm disturbances is thus enhanced. Yet, while acute tachycardia increases ventricular contractility, chronic elevation of heart rate may actually decrease ventricular contractility and precipitate congestive heart failure.[20]

COUNTERBALANCING THE STRESS RESPONSE BY AEROBIC CONDITIONING

Having reviewed the physiological and selected pathological consequences of stress, let us now examine methods by which aerobic exercise conditioning may enhance cardiovascular function and counteract or blunt maladaptive stress responses.

In general, the type of exercise undertaken is determined by the specific conditioning effects desired. Exercise may be prescribed to improve muscular strength, muscular endurance or cardiovascular endurance. The type of exercises best suited for the relief of stress are aerobic or cardiovascular endurance exercises that stimulate near maximal adjustments in the organs of circulation and respiration for relatively extended periods of time. This is the form of exercise (aerobic) referred to exclusively in this discussion. To insure optimal gains in cardiovascular function, the selected physical activities must require moderate contractions of the large muscle groups of the body and must necessitate metabolic adaptation in excess of 70% of the available heart rate range. The concomitant increase in oxygen consumption is sometimes expressed in METS. A MET is defined as the oxygen consumption (energy expenditure at basal conditions; one MET is approximately 3.5 cc of oxygen per kilogram of body weight. It is a useful term for expressing oxygen consumption relative to body mass, thus considering differences in the size of individuals. It is a more useful method in comparing one individual or one group to another than calories consumed per minute, for example.

Exercise as described above must be sustained for 15 to 30 minutes and repeated three to five times per week. Some of the common forms of exercise that enhance cardiovascular function of this variety include running, walking at a brisk pace, swimming and bicycling. Because of the high oxygen consumption of these cardiovascular activities, they are referred to as aerobic exercises. The benefit of aerobic exercise in the physiologic relief of stress depends upon favorable adjustments in (1) maximal oxygen uptake, (2) myocardial and peripheral adaptations, and (3) blood chemistry and fibrinolytic mechanisms.

An improved maximal oxygen uptake consequent to aerobic conditioning depends upon enhanced oxygen transport. The processes that influence oxygen transport are pulmonary function, cardiac output, stroke volume, heart rate and A-VO$_2$ difference. All are improved through aerobic conditioning. A detailed discussion of these can be found elsewhere in the literature.[11] In addition, myocardial oxygen supply and demand are placed in more favorable balance by the diminished heart rate and left ventricular wall tension relative to cardiac output following aerobic conditioning.[10] Furthermore, there is enhanced power function of the heart produced by increased stroke volume and myocardial mechanical efficiency. It is likely that coronary flow is increased on the basis of diminished resistance to coronary flow offered by a decreased rate of development of tension (dP/dt) and enhanced stroke volume, as well as increased time for diastolic flow. These benefits are exclusive of collateral development or dilated coronary vessels.

Chronic tachycardia and elevated aortic pressure were previously cited as maladaptive responses to stress. As noted, exercise conditioning causes a relative bradycardia and decreased arterial pressure for equivalent work levels.[21,22] The increased cardiac output with decreased heart rate accompanying training contributes to a greater stroke volume, improved coronary flow and myocardial efficiency. Unlike the generalized stress response, peripheral vasodilatation during exercise is regional and specific to metabolic need. While both exercise and stress bring about redistribution of peripheral blood flow, they are contrasted by the fact that exercise can reduce systemic vascular resistance, whereas stress increases it.

SELECTION OF PATIENTS FOR EXERCISE CONDITIONING

A physician considering implementation of an exercise program is faced with the individualization of a prescription which has potent therapeutic advantages, yet carries the risk of untoward and potentially fatal side effects. One must know the likelihood of untoward side effects before the implementation of an appropriate exercise program. There are several ways in which objective data can be obtained to assess individual exercise capability. These include the Masters Two-Step Test, bicycle ergometry and treadmill testing, among others. Much evidence suggests that the sensitivity and facility of treadmill testing exceeds that of other usually available, relatively uncomplicated exercise testing methods. My personal preference is for a modification of the Bruce technique. An outline of our protocol for the evaluation of patients follows.

PROTOCOL FOR TREADMILL EXERCISE TESTING*

Three major applications for treadmill testing are (1) detection of myocardial ischemia by evaluation of symptoms and ST segment response; (2) detection, confirmation or follow-up of cardiac arrhythmias; and (3) observation of the functional capacity of the cardiovascular and pulmonary system. The risk of treadmill exercise testing is quite

*Developed by A.D. Forker, M.D. and W. Chambers, M.D. Division of Cardiovascular Medicine, University of Nebraska Medical Center.

minimal, with serious complications occurring in only about one out of 10,000 tests.[23] The patient, however, must sign an informed consent prior to testing.

Contraindications

The test should not be administered if there is any acute or chronic illness that would not allow the patient to exercise comfortably and safely, complete left bundle branch block, left ventricular hypertrophy with "strain", hypokalemia which will create a false positive test, and if any drug is used, particularly digitalis, which would confuse the interpretation of the exercise test. Unstable angina patients should be exercised very carefully, and should be stopped the moment they start having significant pain or a positive ECG. If these patients already have ST segment changes on the resting ECG, the exercise ECG is without value for diagnosing possible myocardial ischemia. In this circumstance, the exercise test provides information only about arrhythmias and the functional capacity of the heart.

Procedure for Performing Exercise Test

The patient should not have eaten for two hours prior to testing to exclude any postprandial ST segment false positive changes. A baseline blood pressure should be taken by the physician, and then the blood pressure should be taken at least once every three minutes while the treadmill test is performed, and again immediately following the test. A supine, standing, and standing plus hyperventilation pre-exercise ECG will be taken. The hyperventilation procedure will exclude any false positive ST segment changes on that basis alone. The most sensitive lead placement is the modified V_5 precordial lead. All twelve leads are placed, but during exercise the V_5 lead will be monitored by computer on the oscilloscope. Every minute during the test, leads V_4, V_5, and V_6 are recorded. A twelve-lead ECG is recorded

BRUCE TREADMILL PROTOCOL			
Stage	Time Per Stage	Speed	Grade
I	3 Minutes	1.7 mph	10%
II	3 Minutes	2.5 mph	12%
III	3 Minutes	3.4 mph	14%
IV	3 Minutes	4.2 mph	16%

Figure 7-1. Bruce treadmill protocol showing Stages I through IV with the time per stage and the corresponding speed and grade.

upon cessation of the exercise test and every minute thereafter. Usually, by six minutes after exercise, the changes that are going to occur have occurred and the monitoring can be stopped. If the test is abnormal, the patient should be monitored until the ECG returns almost to normal and/or the patient is free of symptoms. The patient should not be allowed to support his weight on the hand rails during the exercise test. This would create an isometric response with an inappropriate increase in both heart rate and blood pressure.

The Bruce protocol is utilized for exercise testing. Basically, it starts at 1.7 mph at a 10 percent grade and is increased in speed and incline every three minutes (see Figure 7-1). The target rate for diagnostic exercise testing is at least 85 percent of the patient's age-approximated maximal heart rate capacity (Figure 7-2). This can be estimated by subtracting the patient's age from 200. The maximum difference between normal and ischemic results occurs above exercise heart rates of 150 beats per minute, so this is the minimal level of heart rate response to be achieved. The aim is to keep the patient at or over 85 percent of maximal heart rate capacity for at least three minutes. If this amount of activity is tolerated, we generally allow the person to

PREDICTED MAXIMAL HEART RATES, RECOMMENDED TARGET RATES, and ENDPOINT RATES by AGE for SUBMAXIMAL EXERCISE TESTING.

AGE	20	25	30	35	40	45	50	55	60	65	70	75	80	85
MAXIMAL HEART RATE (UNTRAINED)	197	195	193	191	189	187	184	182	180	178	176	174	172	170
85% of MAXIMAL	167	166	164	162	161	159	156	155	153	151	149	148	146	144
90% of MAXIMAL	177	175	173	172	170	168	166	164	162	160	158	157	155	153

Figure 7-2. Age adjusted heart rates for submaximal exercise testing. The target heart rate for diagnostic exercise testing is 85% of the patient's age adjusted maximal heart rate. The endpoint heart rate is 90% of the patient's age adjusted maximal heart rate.

exercise to his maximal heart rate. After maximal heart rate has been maintained for three minutes, the exercise test can be discontinued at any time. After testing, examine the patient in the supine position after his heart rate begins to slow down for any new signs of gallops or murmurs.

Indications for Stopping Testing

Significant symptoms, significant ventricular arrhythmia, exertional hypotension, ST segment depression greater than 3 mm, ST segment elevation or a systolic blood pressure over 240 mm Hg are all indications for immediately stopping testing.

CRITERIA FOR GRADING THE EXERCISE TEST

The criteria for grading a test as positive for myocardial ischemia are the following: (1) 1.0 mm ST segment depression of a line of down curving nature (not just J point depression); (2) ST segment depression lasting 0.08 seconds; and (3) ST segment depression occurring in three successive beats. The ST segment change should be compared with the preceding PR segment. Although abrupt horizontal 1 to 2 mm ST segment depression is the most commonly utilized parameter for evidence of ischemic heart disease, there are others that deserve consideration. Among the factors that can be considered to denote an abnormal exercise test response, in my view, are the following: failure to elevate blood pressure or a reduction in blood pressure following the onset of exercise, the development of a significant arrhythmia (supraventricular or ventricular), inadequate chronotropic response, the development of typical substernal chest pain, light-headedness or syncope, and pathologic fatigue.

It must be remembered that a positive treadmill test is not specific for obstructive coronary artery disease, it simply suggests myocardial ischemic abnormalities. Among other things, anything that causes an imbalance between myocardial oxygen supply and demand is likely to produce a positive test. In our experience, 85 to 90 percent of the patients with significant obstructive coronary disease will have a positive exercise test. Therefore, there are still 10 to 15 percent of the patients with significant coronary obstructive disease who will be missed by this screening procedure. Good clinical judgment, observation of the patient's pain patterns, the patient's response to exercise, and relief of chest pain with nitroglycerin are helpful in identifying these people. It has recently become clear that the early development of ST segment depression and/or a drop in blood pressure may signal a left main stem coronary arterial obstruction or its equivalent.[24] In such individuals, coronary arteriography is indicated to determine the presence of this potentially fatal lesion. An additional clinical point of concern is the frequent finding of a positive treadmill test in an individual who has no overt subjective evidence of ischemic heart disease. Frequently, a thallium scan will be performed in such individuals. If the radioactive thallium scanning demonstrates ischemia, coronary arteriography is performed. Finally, women are more difficult to exercise because of the artifact created by the left breast. They also have a greater incidence (approaching 30 percent) of false positive ischemic responses.[25]

NON-DIAGNOSTIC USES OF TREADMILL EXERCISE TESTING

In addition to its use as a diagnostic tool, treadmill exercise testing is useful in determining exercise capability. This is helpful in determining safe activities for patients with symptomatic heart disease. It also provides an estimate of the therapeutic effectiveness of an exercise program, as well as medical or surgical treatment.

All treadmill tests present an increasing work load to

the patient by periodic increases in grade and/or treadmill speed. The response to this increasing work load is an increase in oxygen consumption and heart rate. The oxygen consumption is directly related to the work load. The heart rate is linearly related to the work load, but the magnitude of heart rate response depends upon the patient's physical condition. Those in good condition accomplish the treadmill work load at a lower heart rate than those who are sedentary and in poor physical condition. A lower heart rate contributes to a lower myocardial work load and, thus, a lower myocardial oxygen demand.

The Bruce treadmill protocol is most often used. The individual stages with percent grade and treadmill speed are presented in Figure 1. For each stage, the oxygen cost has been previously determined and can be expressed in oxygen consumption per kilogram per minute or in METS.

By using METS, all patients of different weights are normalized by expressing work capacity in multiples of resting metabolic requirements. The oxygen requirement in METS for each stage of the Bruce protocol is presented in Figure 7-3.

The endpoint for the treadmill exercise test is attainment of 90 percent of maximal heart rate or the appearance of previously unrecognized cardiac symptoms or ST depression. Once an exercise test has been terminated for any of the above reasons, the heart rate is noted and the final treadmill stage is matched to the oxygen cost in METS by using Figure 7-3. Figure 7-4 contains the oxygen cost in METS of commonly performed activities. Using the allowable METS from the treadmill test, a sample of allowable activities can be obtained from Figure 4. In addition, it is important that the heart rate during the prescribed activity always stay below the rate at which the treadmill test was stopped. If a patient's physical condition changes or a change in therapy occurs, the patient should be re-tested and new exercise limits established.

To demonstrate how this works, Patient A completes

O₂ Consumption (ml/kg/min)	METS	TREADMILL STAGE (3 minutes per stage)
45.5	13	Stage IV 4.2 mph 16% grade
31.5	9	Stage III 3.4 mph 14% grade
24.5	7	Stage II 2.5 mph 12% grade
17.5	5	Stage I 1.7 mph 10% grade
3.5	1	Rest

Figure 7-3. Oxygen consumption in METS for Bruce treadmill stages. The oxygen cost in METS for the final treadmill stage achieved can be used as a guide for prescribing optimal activities.

Stage I of the Bruce protocol with a heart rate of 120 bpm when angina occurs. Patient B completes Stage III with a heart rate of 140 bpm when significant ST depression occurs. From Figure 3, it is calculated that Patient A can perform activities that require 5 or less METS and Patient B can perform activities that require 7 or less METS. Among other things, Patient A can participate in light carpentry, gardening, walking 3 to 3½ mph, and doubles tennis. Regardless of the activity, the heart rate should not exceed 120 bpm. Patient B can dig ditches, saw hardwood, jog 5 mph, shovel snow, and play touch football. Likewise, regardless of the activity, the heart rate should not exceed 140 bpm.

EXERCISE EVALUATION AFTER AMI

It is often helpful to know whether a patient can achieve minimal exercise testing before release from the hospital following recovery from acute myocardial infarc-

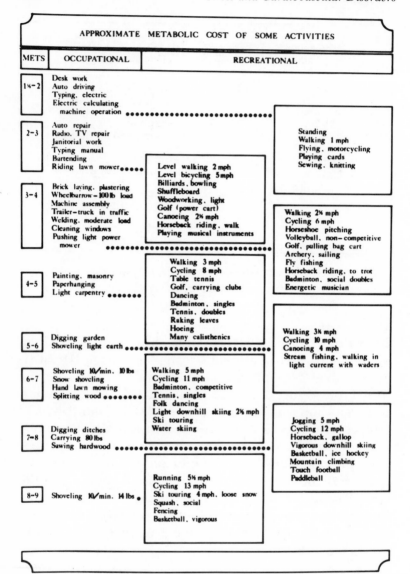

Figure 7-4. The approximate metabolic cost of some occupational and recreational activities. Using the allowable range of METS from Figure 3, a variety of optimal activities can be prescribed for the patient.

tion. In this setting, exercise testing can be accomplished at a very low level, Bruce Stage I or Stage II, depending upon the home situation and the requirements of the patient in that setting. This submaximal testing can involve Holter monitoring instead of treadmill testing. It is surprising how many untoward arrhythmias and other problems can be detected in apparently asymptomatic and uncomplicated patients. Prophylactic antiarrhythmic management, in particular, is greatly assisted by this evaluation.

Submaximal exercise testing before hospital discharge also allows the patient to implement a steady and progressive exercise program. The program, of course, will begin with walking for the first twelve weeks post-infarction. The patient can be taught to measure the pulse and to move at a steadily increasing pace and duration until he reaches 80 percent of his predicted maximum exercise tolerance. It must be remembered to caution patients that the pulse must be taken employing a peripheral radial or brachial artery. Utilization of the carotid pulse may induce carotid sinus syncope.

Another key factor is the selection of exercise appropriate to the individual's life-style. Adherence to an exercise program will be forthcoming if two conditions exist: first, the exercise must be appropriate and handy within the life setting of the individual, and second, the spouse must be enthusiastic in support of the activity. Inappropriate forms of exercise, remoteness of the location for exercise, "the obedience school" approach and, especially, the absence of the spouse's support portend failure. It goes without saying that a knowledge of the patient as an individual is essential to the determination of the form of exercise most likely to offer a lifetime of cardiovascular conditioning. After the first twelve weeks of recovery, a full modified Bruce exercise tolerance test is usually prudent and advisable. In some instances, the date may be moved up to six or eight weeks post-infarction depending upon the clinical circumstances.

GUIDELINES AND PRECAUTIONS FOR EXERCISE
PRESCRIPTION

One of the guidelines for exercise prescription which has been helpful in my experience is the climate in which the individual lives. For those who live in the sun belt, outside activities are reasonable. For those who don't, a form of exercise such as stationary bicycle riding can be offered as an option to walking, jogging or cycling. For many who live in climates which have extremes of heat or cold, the enclosed shopping mall has been an excellent alternative to the more restrictive in-house stationary bicycle exercise. For maximum benefit, exercise must be consistent without interruption for a period of 20 to 40 minutes, 3 to 5 times per week.

Group programs offer a variety of activities, usually under careful supervision with a CPR-trained nurse, defibrillator and/or resuscitative team in attendance. Supervised programs in rural communities are less available and, therefore, special considerations must be made on this basis.

Under all circumstances, patients should start slowly. Many sedentary individuals, especially those recovering from acute myocardial infarction, attempt to undo years of inactivity within a few days or weeks. This misguided enthusiasm may lead to recurrent ischemic episodes, muscle cramps, march fractures, acute gout, increased upper respiratory infection and a host of other cardiovascular or orthopedic complications. This would be enough to permanently demoralize a Hercules (Figure 7-5). Undoubtedly, many such individuals have formed the charter membership of Athletics Anonymous, a group who in total frustration have organized in the same fashion as Alcoholics Anonymous. At the first urge to exercise, they call their buddy who immediately talks them out of it.

Thus, the "starter program" is extremely important and may require one to four weeks of very gradual increase

COMPLICATIONS of JOGGING

MUSCULOSKELETAL
 March Fracture, Plantar
 Fasciitis, Hallux Rigidus,
 Ligamental Strain,
 Tendinitis, Muscle Rupture,
 Stress Fracture, Shin
 Splints, Bursitis, Periostitis,
 Sinovial Effusion, Hemar-
 throsis of Ankle, Patellar
 Chondromalacia,
 Exacerbation of Back Pain

ABDOMINAL
 Inguinal Hernia,
 Hemorrhoids, Hiatal Hernia

CUTANEOUS
 Corns, Calluses, Blisters,
 Petechial Hemorrhage of
 Ankle

RENAL
 Pseudonephritis

PULMONARY
 Asthma Attacks, Exacerba-
 tion of Upper Respiratory
 Illness, Deep Inhalation of
 Smog

CARDIOVASCULAR
 Sudden Cardiac Death,
 Myocardial Infarction,
 Arrhythmias, Stroke,
 Precipitation of Heart
 Failure

NEUROLOGIC/
PSYCHOLOGIC
 Subarachnoid Hemorrhage,
 Depression after
 Discontinuance

FLUID AND ELECTROLYTES
 Fluid Loss, Temperature
 Elevation, Heat Stroke,
 Electrolyte Disturbance

Figure 7-5. Potential complications of jogging. Adapted from M.S. Hoffman.[26]

from slow to brisk walking before more intense forms of exercise can be implemented. Walking is often disdained, but is especially valuable for the elderly who may have no need or desire to join the geriatric jocks, and who may enjoy the social aspects of walking with the spouse at a brisk pace. Granted, it takes longer to accomplish cardiovascular conditioning with walking and the level of conditioning is not that associated with more strenuous forms of exercise. It is, however, an appropriate form of exercise which fulfills many of the hemodynamic and humanistic needs of the individual.

A period of warm-up and cool-down is essential for individuals who participate in exercise programs. Abrupt implementation or discontinuance of exercise is frequently associated with undesirable cardiovascular responses. In addition, the dress should be appropriate both to the activity and to the weather. Proper footwear is imperative, especially for those who choose to jog. A good quality running shoe, in such instances, is essential and far more satisfactory in the prevention of orthopedic disasters than the frequently employed flat-soled tennis shoe. In extremes of climate, one should avoid plastic or rubber sweat suits which produce excessive heat loads and sweating. This is especially important in high risk patients who should avoid exercising outdoors in extremes of temperature.

The physician must assist the patient in selecting an appropriate time for exercise. Although there is much individualization in this regard, it is advantageous to avoid exercise for at least one hour after meals owing to the redistribution of blood flow.

One of the potentially fatal mistakes that is made in many instances in exercise programs is the return to the same level of physical activity following a period of illness or layoff. It is possible to decondition a fully conditioned system in as little as one to three weeks subsequent to the cessation of exercise conditioning.[27] Obviously, resuming the same workload after such a period represents a severe hazard. A good rule of thumb has been offered by Dehn and Mullins: "Have your patient decrease one work level for every workout missed and then *gradually* work back to the previous work level."[28]

It is also important to avoid competitive exercise or so-called "all out" efforts. Often those who become interested and active in exercise programs are basically competitive individuals. It is also known that competitors who become leading athletes are those who are most capable of suppressing pain. Indeed, the winning of any race, marathon or otherwise, requires considerable ability to deny great physical discomfort. For the patient with ischemic heart disease, this denial can be fatal, since chest pain is one of the important warning systems. In a competitive setting, such an individual may unfortunately deny important symptoms, thereby risking arrhythmias, cardiovascular complications and even death.

It is extremely important also to advise patients against exercising during periods of illness. Certain illnesses deplete body fluids, and in a state of dehydration the individual is well known to be predisposed to arrhythmias. One should caution patients against a hot shower immediately following exercise. The external heat load offered from hot showers, steam baths, saunas or other such techniques is associated with a rapid fall in peripheral resistance and blood pressure. The latter can induce a sudden fall in coronary flow, setting the stage for arrhythmias. The sauna offers the additional risk of external heat load and its hemodynamic effects followed by the sudden cold with remarkable opposing hemodynamic effects. The hazard of the extreme physiologic changes associated with such techniques is documented by detailed Finnish studies reporting the sauna as the place associated with the highest incidence of sudden death of any location in Finland.[29]

After exercise, patients should be allowed a period to cool off for at least 20 minutes before taking a shower, which at best should be lukewarm, neither hot nor ice cold.

SUMMARY

In summary, the goal of an exercise program is to improve the quality of the individual's life. There is only suggestive evidence to indicate that exercise programs, beginning in youth or following infarction, prolong life. Exercise can improve the quality of life, increase work capacity at the lowest possible myocardial oxygen cost, reduce the stress on the cardiovascular system, and perhaps even facilitate the handling of emotional stress as well. However, preliminary results after two years from the Ontario Exercise-Heart Collaborative Study[30] report a higher incidence of reinfarction in the high intensity group (32 infarcts, N = 386) than in the low intensity exercise group (22 infarcts, N = 365). Although these differences are not statistically significant, it appears that exercise conditioning does not contribute to increased longevity.

Before implementing such exercise programs, one must know one's patient as an individual, including his habits and patterns and his exercise capability. This is accomplished preferably by treadmill testing, and is important in all cases, but especially in the post-infarction patient or in the patient with hypertensive cardiovascular disease. In the former, one must know the limits to which a potentially ischemic heart can be pushed; in the latter, a hypertensive patient may be an undetected ischemic patient or may hyperreact in an exercise setting. When balanced with a knowledge of the individual, his life-style, and his potential to perform, it is likely that the goal of adherence will be better achieved. Both initial and continuing evaluation and motivation are essential to the effectiveness of exercise conditioning and the avoidance of unnecessary and untoward complications.

REFERENCES

1. Choquette, G., and Ferguson, R.J.: Blood pressure reduction in "borderline" hypertensives following physical training. *Canadian Med. Assoc. J.* **108**:699-703, 1973.
2. Chanutin, A., and Curnish, R.R.: Effect of organic and inorganic phosphates on the oxygen equilibrium of human erythrocytes. *Arch. Biochem. Biophys.* **121**:96-102, 1967.

3. Åkeson, Å., Biörck, G., and Simon, R.M.: On the content of myoglobin in human muscles. *Acta Med. Scand.* **183**:307, 1968.

4. Biörck, G.: Hematin compounds in mammalian heart and skeletal msucle. *Amer. Heart J.* **52**:624, 1956.

5. Barmeyer, J.: Physical activity and coronary collateral development. In V. Manninen and P.I. Halonen (Eds): *Physical Activity and Coronary Heart Disease, Advances in Cardiology,* Volume 18. Basel: S. Karger A.G., 1976, pp. 104-112.

6. Gregg, D.E., and Fisher, L.C.: Blood supply to the heart. In W.E. Hamilton and P. Dow (Eds.): *Handbook of Physiology,* Volume 2. Washington, D.C.: American Physiological Society, 1963.

7. Burt, J.J., and Jackson, R.: Coronary collateral development. *J. Sportmed.* **5**:203, 1965.

8. Kaplinsky, E., Hood, W.B., McCarthy, B., et al: Effect of physical training in dogs with coronary artery ligation. *Circulation* **37**:556-565, 1968.

9. Baroldi, G.: Personal communication. November, 1976.

10. Eliot, R.S., Forker, A.D., and Robertson, R.J.: Aerobic exercise as a therapeutic modality in the relief of stress. In V Manninen and P.I. Halonen (Eds.): *Physical Activity and Coronary Heart Disease, Advances in Cardiology,* Volume 18. Basel: S. Karger A.G., 1976, pp. 231-242.

11. Åstrand, P.O., and Rodahl, K.: *Textbook of Work Physiology.* New York: McGraw-Hill, 1970, p. 173.

12. Mitchell, J.H., and Wildenthal, K.: Static (isometric) exercise and the heart: Physiological and clinical considerations. *Annual Review Med.* **25**:369, 1974.

13. Mullins, C.B., and Bloomqvist, G.: Isometric exercise and the cardiac patient. *Texas Med.* **69**:53, 1973.

14. Atkins, J.M., Matthews, O.A., Bloomqvist, C.G., and Mullins, C.B.: Incidence of arrhythmias induced by isometric and dynamic exercise. *Brit. Heart J.* **38**:465-471, 1976.

15. Workshop IV: Emotional stress and coronary artery disease. *J. South Carolina Med. Assoc.* (Supplement) **72**:88-95, 1976.

16. Abrahams, V.C., Hilton, S.M., and Brozyna, A.W.: The role of active muscle vasodilatation in the alerting stage of the

defense reaction. *J. Physiol. (London)* **171**:189-202, 1964.

17. Sokoloff, L., Mangold, R., Wechsler, R.L., et al: The effect of mental arithmetic on cerebral circulation and metabolism. *J. Clin. Invest.* **34**:1011-1108, 1955.

18. Gilmore, J.P., and Gerlings, E.D.: Influence of developed tension on myocardial potassium balance in the dog heart. *Circ. Res.* **22**:769-775, 1968.

19. Maling, H.M., and Highman, B.: Exaggerated ventricular arrhythmias and myocardial fatty changes after large doses of norepinephrine and epinephrine in unanesthetized dogs. *Amer. J. Physiol.* **194**:590-596, 1958.

20. Coleman, H.N., Taylor, R.R., Pool, P.E., et al: Congestive heart failure following chronic tachycardia. *Amer. Heart J.* **81**:790-798, 1971.

21. Boyer, J.: Effects of chronic exercise on cardiovascular function. In H.H. Clarke (Ed.): *Physical Fitness Research Digest.* Washington, D.C.: President's Council on Physical Fitness and Sports, Series 2, No. 3, 1972.

22. Clausen, J.P., and Trap-Jensen, J.: Effects of training on the distribution of cardiac output in patients with coronary artery disease. *Circulation* **42**:611-624, 1970.

23. Naughton, J.P., Hellerston, H.K., and Mohler, I.C.: *Exercise Testing and Training in Coronary Heart Disease.* New York: Academic Press, 1973.

24. Kleiner, J.P., Boland, M.J., and Brundage, B.H.: The markedly positive stress test. Is it an indicator of left main coronary disease? *Circulation* **54**: Supplement II:206, 1976 (abstract).

25. Ellestad, M., Savitz, S., Bergdall, D., and Teske, J.: The false positive stress test: Multivariate analysis of 215 subjects with hemodynamic, angiographic, and clinical data. *Amer. J. Cardiol.* **40**:681-685, 1977.

26. Hoffman, M.S.: Complications of jogging. *American College of Cardiology Extended Learning* (ACCEL tape) 10, Number 6, June, 1978.

27. Saltin, B., Bloomqvist, G., Mitchell, J.H., et al: Response to exercise after bed rest and after training: A longitudinal study of adaptive changes in oxygen transport and body composition. *Circulation* **38**: Supplement VII:1-78, 1968.

28. Dehn, M.M., and Mullins, C.B.: Physiologic effects and importance of exercise in patients with coronary artery disease. *Cardiovasc. Med.* **2**:365-387, 1977.

29. Luurila, O.: Cardiac arrhythmias, sudden death, and Finnish sauna bath. In V. Manninen and P.I. Halonen (Eds.): *Advances in Cardiology*, Volume 25. Basel: S. Karger A.G. 1978, pp. 73-81.

30. Rechnitzer, P.: Exercise in the Post Coronary Patient: Effects of Training on Re-infarction and Recurrence. Presentation at the 25th Annual Meeting of the American College of Sports Medicine. Washington, D.C., May, 1978.

CHAPTER 8

FAMILY LIFE

The family's role today ranges from a cause of stress to a powerful and preserving support system buttressed against it. Often the clinician must determine what role the family plays in his patient's life. To accomplish this, it may occasionally be necessary to utilize the talents of family counselors. The variety of techniques available in family counseling is complex and beyond the scope of this text, yet it is the physician's domain to recognize the need for these services and to monitor their progress. For these reasons, it seems important to present a perspective of family life in today's world.

It is helpful to begin by reviewing the metamorphosis of the family in western society in recent history. Since the inception of civilization, the family fabric has been woven with two basic threads: love and mutual assistance. The extended family provided education, protection, health care, and looked after its aged members. These original inherent functions of the family are now being provided by the community and supported by private, state, or federal agencies. Today, the family no longer is the focal point for the education of children or the teaching of a craft. Vocational skills were previously passed from father to son within the family. Currently, they have become the responsibility of educational institutions capable of teaching the unique and diverse requirements basic to the multivocational job market of today.

Formerly, the extended family gathered in time of internal and external danger to protect its members, a role now provided to a great extent by police and firemen locally, and by the armed forces nationally. The need for sustenance in periods of sickness was provided by non-hospital sources in the form of folk medicine or a grand-mother, aunt, cousin, or some other relative. Family responsibility also shrank inversely with the advent of insurance policies, Social Security checks, and a variety of state and federal agencies.

With the American industrial revolution came the requirement for geographic relocation of family members in order to find gainful employment. The family no longer clustered around a particular trade in a particular geographic area. Instead, it became fragmented and it moved, becoming scattered into urban isolation. The nuclear family was usually the only intact recognizable residual. Thus, the extended American family of the past has been slimmed and trimmed in current terms to a small, detached nuclear unit composed of a husband, wife, and unmarried children. Biological interactions based on consanguinity or "kinship" have largely disappeared; they dissolved into Sunday gatherings at first, later they diminished to include only holidays, weddings or funerals. Ironically, nowadays the funeral is often the only gathering of the extended kinship group.

The roles of family members have changed dramatically in a dynamic changing world with its diversity of experiences and resultant cultural shock. Stress increasingly prevails with the gradual disappearance of accepted and traditional patterns of behavior. Today, stress pervades all levels and periods of family life. First, marital stress between husband and wife has become more evident as the wife's changing role has allowed her to become less timid, dependent, subservient and "obedient" as she had earlier promised in her marriage vows. It remains true that a majority of women seek marriage in some form, but desire ever smaller family units, or perhaps no children at all. This in itself can induce stress because of pre-existing cultural designs for children as a natural part of the family unit. For parents and hopeful grandparents of an earlier traditional molding, there is often disappointment and outright hostility directed at married couples, who are childless by choice.

Relationships also become strained as children arrive and bring new responsibilities, time demands, and conflicts into focus. Modern children rarely succumb to the "being seen but not heard" behavior of the past. They no longer appear to be tiny adults. More often they display sibling rivalry as an increasingly frequent sign of our times.

Women today frequently find great social and economic pressure for utilizing their educational, business, and professional capabilities. Fulfillment may not be found in managing a household, raising children or performing the classic role of nurture and support. It must be pointed out that although many appear to prefer the latter role, they are often scorned by those who feel such women are succumbing to the male chauvinists of our times. Many women argue that they have more to offer than the maternal and sexual roles of the past. Here, too, social pressures create ambivalence, anxiety, and stress in today's women.

It is certainly the woman who tries to be all things to all people at all times who is most stressed. This "woman for all seasons" seeks identity not only in the nurture and support roles, but also in the world of business. For her, there is often double identity, double the work, and double the stress. Consequently, she is rarely at peace with her ambivalence.

The two remaining family threads are those of love and mutual assistance. Today, a person moves from his family of birth to his family of procreation, at least overtly, on the basis of love. Love and mutual support, therefore, are often the only adhesives that glue the contemporary family together. When these basic features are viewed along with the increasing independence sought by all family members, it becomes apparent that a person's total needs can no longer be met by the nuclear family. Indeed, the contemporary conflicts between seeking independence and meeting dependency needs place increasing pressure on family structure and cohesiveness.

The family of the past was thus bound together by residence and income, and served as the most formative and fundamental group to which any person could belong. Today, the family is perpetuated more by happenstance and accident than by the formulation and pursuit of tradition. As these tangible dimensions fade, there is a reciprocal enhancement of the more intangible needs less related to survival. These include, for example, income in case of death, education, increased intimacy, better communication skills and less rigidity.

It is clearly a concern that no society has ever survived without the family. Certainly the pioneer family of the past finds very little opportunity for further development today. Indeed, many contemporary business and professional people reject the family as an anachronistic hobby, a deterrent, or at best a luxury of questionable utility. Daily, we find more individuals who literally live at their place of business, maintaining little, if any, identity with their nuclear family or the extended family unit of the past.

A logical consequence is to be found in the increase in couples who either live together, have contract marriages or no formal legal relationships. For many, these relationships were formed for the purposes of sharing costs, satisfying basic physiologic needs, obtaining mutual emotional support, and reducing dependency or interdependency. In this manner, more time is made available to direct attention and energy toward the ever-increasing demands of the business and professional world.

A word must be said about the roles that inflation and the Internal Revenue Service have played in setting the stage for these new living arrangements. Cost has altered morality in accordance with today's "Golden Rule". That is, he who has the gold makes the rule. When inflation outdistances available gold, people combine resources to reach common objectives. Today, the Internal Revenue Service offers the incentive of larger deductions for those who live together without marriage. These incentives even extend into Social Security benefits. In this regard, President Carter expressed some of his best Baptist concerns about the immorality fostered by such systems. Nevertheless, monetary reward remains a potent motivational force in the new "family" structures.

Some of the current experiments give evidence of successfully meeting the mutual needs of the experimentors. Others that were originally cults have become an accepted part of new interdependency relationships in a broadened family setting. The successful ones usually contain the basic ingredients of love and mutual support.

Even in its contemporary or future form, the new family remains a fundamental support system in times of stress. Often it is the critical factor in coping with crises and with facilitating rehabilitation thereafter. Thus, an important role of the practitioner is to determine what form of relationship exists, and whether the support systems therein will assist in or deter from achieving preventive or rehabilitative goals.

BEHAVIOR IN VARIOUS FAMILY SETTINGS

In times of disaster, such as a major cardiovascular illness, new and unique pressures are applied to the family unit, whatever its makeup. Here, basic human needs for emotional support are required from some source. In this setting, the family can be a major and potent therapeutic tool in the alleviation of additional stress. Yet, at these times there is often a temporary or permanent reversal of dominant marital roles when income is lost or threatened. These major changes in lifestyle often immobilize or deter family members from individual and mutual goals. The contemporary family in transition thus finds it difficult to function as a buttress against stress when it experiences the additional turmoil of illness in a key member.

Detectable behaviors at this time vary, but are engrafted on old established patterns. Some of these can be viewed as common or even categorical. Although interrelationships are different, they often share common features. The categories described below are indistinct and blurred with many overlapping boundaries. They are offered only as guidelines or landmarks.

The first such example is the *wife whose identity is entirely wrapped up in her husband.* For this woman, her husband's illness may evoke anger, in that her own career goals, identity and abilities may have been side-tracked or suppressed and are now sacrificed by his current illness. The abandonment of her hopes, identity and future subsequent to such illness may be blamed on her husband. This is frequently followed by guilt, and a vicious cycle develops.

Another and more acceptable form of dependency is often displayed in blue collar workers. Here, *male dominance* is an accepted traditional role, well understood, and conforming with pioneer family guidelines. Often, in this setting, the wife is a dependent but equal partner who is more easily mobilized in a support sense as it represents no real conflict.

A third variety is the *wife dominated,* "mother makes it right" category. When this husband becomes ill, a transient increase in his dependence can usually be well tolerated. Temporary encouragement of this behavior can be a useful therapeutic measure when this relationship exists. Should the wife become ill, however, a conflict usually arises in view of the dependency needs of the husband which are no longer met by his stricken spouse.

Another marital relationship is the narcissistic or hysterical *"yes dear" wife,* who is intellectually superficial and incapable of playing a genuine supportive role. Very often, such a wife has acquired an obsessive, compulsive husband as a matter of necessity. Illness for this husband can be disastrous, since the wife is often incapable of offering emotional support to her stricken husband. In the opposite setting, an obsessive, compulsive husband can be very effective in patching up the ego of a more hysterical wife. In this instance, the key is reassurance from the husband that the wife's attractiveness has been unblemished by the illness.

In all of these circumstances, it is important to observe and identify the dynamics of these relationships. For example, is it the victim or the spouse who "makes it happen" or who "lets it happen"? During the shock of illness, this may be difficult to detect. Interviewing other family members or friends can often be helpful here. It is well to keep in mind that few partnerships are truly equal.

COUNSELING OPTIONS

When conflicts are found, a variety of counseling and support systems can be offered by the practitioner. These obviously may include other members of the family, friends, neighbors or professionals. Yet, in the latter category, the family physician is the key. Clinical psychologists and social workers are often helpful also. Psychiatric intervention is to be reserved for more serious and complicated problems. When appropriate, the clergy are often of great benefit.

From the previous discussion, it is apparent that the family is a complex and fragile unit in transition in a rapidly changing world, lacking resilience, easily broken and resisting restoration. Revamping family lifestyles overnight is unlikely. It can be hoped, however, that if successful living arrangements existed prior to the illness, they will be maintained and supportive.

The next decade will be crammed with a variety of experiments in family living arrangements engrafted upon the pragmatic principles of trial and error. The effective-

ness of the astute clinician can be greatly aided by an understanding of his patient's unique living arrangement, his
available support systems and his family goals. This understanding, insight and guidance is the key to restoring and
rehabilitating any member to a better quality, and perhaps
even a better quantity, of life.

CHAPTER 9

REHABILITATION AND PREVENTION

It has been estimated that there are 600,000 graduates of coronary care units each year. With the help of various types of rehabilitation programs, these people can again be active members of society. Rehabilitation is a process that also follows surgical interventive procedures, such as saphenous vein bypass grafting. Completion of operations for ischemic heart disease without rehabilitation is an incomplete victory. Prevention, however, is a different matter, since cause remains a multifactorial mystery. Attempts to develop awareness, motivation and adherence for preventive programs remain difficult and disappointing. Unfortunately, modification of behavior often requires a powerful insult which awakens insight. Insight is fundamental to the implementation of any behavior modification. Accordingly, this chapter will emphasize rehabilitation. In some instances, the statements on rehabilitation parallel goals for prevention. It will be recalled that prevention is a dream and not a reality at this time. Much has been learned about rehabilitation and I will concentrate on new and useful information, practical in most clinical settings.

REHABILITATION

First we must establish goals to be accomplished for rehabilitation, not only for the patient but also for his family. These include:
1. acceptance of the disease;

2. knowledge of the disease, thereby permitting the patient to make better decisions for his future;
3. emotional support;
4. sustained adherence;
5. reaching the optimal functional level.

Now that the operation and effect of coronary care units is well understood, it can clearly be indicated that the nurse's role in the management of acute myocardial infarction is well established. Reduction of mortality from potentially fatal arrhythmias has been largely the result of sophisticated critical care nursing. It is now almost socially unacceptable to expire as a result of a cardiac arrhythmia. The usual mode of terminal exodus in a coronary care unit at this writing involves power failure secondary to extensive myocardial necrosis. One of the major roles of the nursing staff in conjunction with the physician today should be that of rehabilitation. Certainly, the nurse has the greatest opportunity to observe the patient, establish rapport and interact to initiate and maintain the momentum of rehabilitation.

The first question to be asked after the emergency has passed is, "Why now?" What circumstances could have contributed to the acute event? Is the infarction purely the end result of uncontrolled risk factors such as cholesterol, smoking, obesity, diabetes or hypertension? Are there some additional precipitating factors, such as loss of a spouse, trouble with the boss, marital difficulties and the like? Usually, patients will not volunteer this information. They may be stoic or lack insight, therefore these questions must be asked.

Psychiatric difficulties frequently go unnoticed, yet are reported in from 30 to 70 percent of coronary care unit patients.[1] Usually they are not severe. The commonest difficulty is anxiety resulting from the events surrounding the immediate threat to life. This period should not extend beyond 24 to 48 hours. It is often reassuring to the patient to indicate after the 24 hour period that more heart attack victims die within the first 24 hours than within the next five years. Every reader or television viewer has been sensitized to the risk of chest pain, its complications and potentially fatal outcome. The disease has also touched nearly every family in the industrialized world. Thus, the fear of the event itself is usually superimposed upon an overburdened myocardium.

The control of anxiety is often subtle. Well trained, concerned nursing and medical staffs often, by their manner alone, allay anxiety. A quiet atmosphere is essential to establishing confidence and reducing anxiety. It has been my misfortune to visit, and occasionally to work in, coronary care facilities which more closely approximated a macabre Disney World atmosphere than the quiet, secure, competent setting so essential to managing the first phase of infarction.

Each institution must decide what is an adequate, but not excessive, number of people who will reassure (but not overdo); what is an appropriate amount of technical equipment, rather than an electronic Taj Mahal; and what is the most conducive atmosphere to be established. To my mind, invasive studies and monitoring devices should only be employed in instances where they significantly influence management, and should be undertaken with the least possible discomfort to the patient. In addition to minimizing anxiety, simplicity also offers safety, especially when equipment is used infrequently. There is a natural tendency for techniques to become rusty between uses.

Optimal medication is tantamount to gaining the attention of the patient in order that rehabilitation can be initiated after the first 24 hours of establishing initial rapport. In my experience, diazepam is the agent of choice when anxiety is present, as it tends to assist the aforementioned measures. When pain is present, it, too, can induce a malignant cycle of anxiety. Accordingly, analgesia, preferably with morphine, is essential until such a time that pain is no longer a problem. The mere presence of pain must imply to any rational patient that the situation remains uncontrolled. Most patients also fear the near total loss of control, the essential dependence upon others and the loss of autonomy and options.

Within the first 24 to 48 hours, the staff has achieved rapport with the new patient and the anxiety has been resolved. Thereafter, it is almost a rule of thumb that depression sets in.[2] This form of depression usually involves reality considerations by the patient. There is the threat to autonomy, lifestyle, and routine added to the threat of enforced dependence. The latter is already reenforced by the need to be served, monitored and observed in a dependent fashion quite foreign to usual activity. The depression may also represent a late phase of the initial denial common in acute myocardial infarction. The reality sets in that "I could have died," adding further dimension to the helpless feeling. There is often a strong component of anger at the near total loss of control of one's life or environment. Clearly, this is usually a secondary depression in acute myocardial infarction and is almost always a self-limited circumscribed event. It can be dispatched with greater speed by demonstrating to the patient appropriate evidence of his rehabilitative potential.

It must be assumed that almost all graduates of coronary care units can be rehabilitated to some degree. The majority will and can return to an almost normal lifestyle, or at least to whatever state pre-existed the infarction. This is particularly true in view of the low energy requirements (METS) for most occupations in the industrialized world. Others can return to a modified lifestyle with appropriate adjustments. Some may be helped by surgical intervention. Only a minority are so disabled as to be considered eligible only for custodial care.

The alert staff reminds itself that depression is easily overlooked. It may present as sleep disturbances, pathologic fatigue, or anorexia. A major part of rehabilitation and anti-depressive therapy is direct, constructive information. It is essential to recognize that the patient's ability to concentrate will be limited for the first few days. Informational input, therefore, should be carefully considered, uniform, succinct, and in terms fully understood by the patient. Instruction should be directed toward programmed steps in rehabilitation.

As a teaching adjunct, we have developed a series of audiovisual tapes designed for patient education and rehabilitation, the Heartline to Health series.* These tapes inform the patient about the following topics: (1) What You Should Know About Your Heart; (2) The Risks You Take; (3) High Blood Pressure; (4) Smoke Gets in Your Eyes and Lungs and Heart; (5) Diabetes and Heart Disease; (6) Are You Under Stress; (7) How to Handle Today's Stress; (8) Exercise for Health; (9) Diet, You Can Do It; (10) Good Eating Habits; (11) Menus and Appetites; (12) Checking Out Your Heart; (13) Life After the Attack; and (14) Heart Health: A Family Affair.

Each videocassette tape is approximately 15 to 20 minutes in length. It has the advantage that it can easily be replayed and can be controlled by the patient. In other words, he can replay it until the information is clear. The physician and nursing staff are saved the repetitious task of informing and re-informing. Standard information is frequently given in a different fashion and state of completeness by a variety of staff members on alternate days to patients with relatively similar conditions. The uniformity of carefully edited information is important and valuable; yet appropriate individualization of this standard information must be provided by medical staff familiar with the unique nature of the patient's condition.

It is also extremely important for the staff to explain each piece of equipment that is applied and why it is being

---

*Heartline to Health color videocassette series. Developed by the Cardiovascular Center of the University of Nebraska. Originally broadcast on Nebraska ETV network.

applied. A positive attitude of the staff with genuine concern (but not overconcern) creates the delicate balance fundamental to relieving anxiety, allaying depression, and
motivating rehabilitative efforts.

On completion of the first phase of acute myocardial
infarction, the medical and nursing staff should have
formed a strong rapport with the patient, determined who
he is, where he is coming from and where he can go as a total
psychobiologic unit. Knowledge of his cardiac output, the
presence or absence of arrhythmias, blood pressure, blood
cholesterol level and cardiomegaly are helpful bits of technical information contributing to a comprehensive approach to rehabilitative care. By this time, the relationship
between the spouse and the family or close friends should
be apparent (see Chapter 8 for more information). If
the momentum of rehabilitation is to be maintained, the
family or close friends as well as those who have the nursing
responsibility in the next phase of care must be kept informed.

Transfer out of the coronary care unit represents a loss
to the patient who already has experienced a severe loss.
This move may imply to the patient a loss of attention,
rapport, security, and, in a sense, a loss of identity, which is
already a problem to the victim of acute myocardial infarction. Inattention to these details can lead to a disruptive
transfer with the exacerbation of anxiety, depression and
other complications. If not quickly recognized, they can
lead to further cardiovascular or psychological complications. This anxiety and depression may be accompanied by
elevations of urinary catecholamines during the time immediately following transfer to intermediate care facilities.[3]
The primary goal for the intermediate staff, then, is establishing rapport and offering further reassurance by demonstration of the knowledge gained from the coronary care
unit staff. Too often, the patient feels he has been
"dumped" into the hands of those less informed and less
concerned.

To aid in transition, mild tranquilization may be necessary, and I have found diazepam to be helpful. In my experience, when sleep is a problem, flurazepam is preferred. The latter has been effective and does not appear to interfere with REM sleep, important in the maintenance of psychological adjustment.

It is recognized that the majority of hospitals at this time do not have intermediate care units as such. More often, the coronary care unit graduate is transferred to a ward where nurses have general as well as intermediate coronary care responsibilities. It is to be re-emphasized that all information gained in the coronary care unit must be shared with those in charge of the intermediate phase of rehabilitation. Transition is also smoothed by introducing the intermediate care staff a day or two before the patient leaves the coronary care unit. When transfer is accomplished in this fashion, it is often viewed by the patient as tangible evidence of improvement. This is reenforced by increased activity, less attention or rigid control and a little more autonomy. Equally, there is often great value in the 'esprit de corps' established by association with other patients who have progressed further than the immediate coronary care unit graduate.

Prior to discharge from the hospital, a full knowledge of the home situation is essential for successful rehabilitation. Among the most critical factors is how the spouse views the myocardial infarction. Frequently, the spouse will display anger directed at the infarction or its victim on the basis that marital goals have not yet been achieved and that they may be postponed or permanently lost through disability or death. Sometimes the victim of an acute myocardial infarction is an aggressive, so-called type A, S.O.B. husband who for years has suppressed his wife's individuality. Here the wife's anger may develop on a different basis. If this type of husband has been physically weakened and rendered unable to return to his previous lifestyle, the wife may become dominant, domineering or downright hostile. This form of role reversal can be a destructive experience for the husband, who then may have no choice but to assume a dependent relationship governed by punitive or retaliative intents. In this setting, often the physician and nursing staff and the clergy can work together to help the couple. Once the problem is recognized, ventilation sessions for the spouse are useful for discharging years of pent-up or suppressed hostility.

Despite all the aforementioned efforts, depression may set in again following hospitalization. The major contributing factors include genuine weakness, fatigue, the sense of dependency and enforced changes in lifestyle. It is important to inform the patient that weakness and fatigue are normally expected when bed rest continues past four or five days. This weakness and fatigue may not result from weakness of the heart but simply an untuning of the autonomic nervous system, quite within normal expectations. It should be emphasized that this period of dependency is brief and the reward for adherence to medical and lifestyle regimens is more independence. The patient should recognize that if the previous lifestyle was complete and satisfactory, it is unlikely it would have contributed to the patient's illness. Accordingly, picking appropriate priorities and readjusting lifestyles are essential. These must be blended with appropriate reward systems that are in balance with social and employment obligations. When accomplished, they can enhance the quality of life.

It is not unusual for the patient to experience sleep disorders on returning home. Many of these are related to the aforementioned anxieties and concerns. The loss of supervision, monitoring and potential resuscitative techniques represents a loss of security which can, and often does, temporarily frighten patients. Time itself, aided by family support, usually heals that wound.

Physical conditioning is fundamental to the retraining of the patient. A well designed staging process for the patient with acute myocardial infarction has been developed by Nanette K. Wenger of Emory University.[4] Since these studies have been well thought out and evaluated in large numbers of patients, they form a theme upon which individual variations can be designed (Figure 9-1). After progressing through the inhospital rehabilitation program, I have found it useful to employ heart rate as a guide to cardiac work and to teach patients to monitor their heart rate when increasing their levels of activity. Most patients don't understand that it is the rate at which the heart is working, rather than that at which the body is working, that is important (see Chapter 7 for further details). It is obvious that exercise conditioning must be suited to the individual's lifestyle and must progress gradually over a period of three months before full activity is achieved. Much individualization is essential here, and the activities must be spelled out very carefully. In my view, it is essential to obtain Holter monitoring in the hospital prior to discharge. This procedure will disclose unforeseen, potentially fatal cardiac arrhythmias at levels of exercise to be sustained for the first few weeks following discharge. This preview sets the stage for subsequent careful treadmill testing. The latter might be cautiously conducted six weeks following acute myocardial infarction. Obviously, it will not be done to competitive or maximum Bruce stages. Instead, the goal is to provide guidelines for the physician with regard to levels of activity at safe heart rates without untoward changes in blood pressure, fatigue, level of consciousness or in the electrocardiogram. The aforementioned components are frequently overlooked, yet extremely important in the prediction of potential complications.

On re-entering the home situation, a call from the physician or from the nurse is frequently well received and extremely important in getting feedback for further rehabilitative efforts. What the patient says his home life is and what is viewed on the home visit may be two distinctly different pictures. In this instance, the well trained, perceptive nurse plays an extremely important role on what ap-

Step	Exercise	Care Activities	Other Activities
1	Passive range of motion exercise to extremities *(5 times each)*, active plantar and dorsiflexion of ankles *(several times/day)*	Feeding self *(head of bed at 45° angle, trunk and arms supported by over-bed table)*	Initial interview, brief description of program
2	AS ABOVE	Feeding self, partial morning care in bed, dangle legs on side of bed *(1 time)*	Light activity such as reading
3	Active assisted exercise: shoulder flexion; elbow flexion and extension; hip flexion, extension, and rotation; knee flexion and extension; rotate feet. *(4-times each)*	Sitting in chair for short periods (2 times/day), bathe whole body, use bedside commode	More detailed explanation of program, light activity continued

Figure 9-1. *An example of a step-wise progression of various activities suitable for initiating rehabilitation of the patient with acute myocardial infarction. Adapted from N.K. Wenger.*[4]

pears to be a simple and straightforward social visit. The visit also provides opportunities for the patient to ask questions in a comfortable setting after a trial period at home. These questions might not emerge in a harried office visit. This follow-through management can be extremely effective in allaying anxiety and depression, thereby enhancing the effectiveness of the rehabilitative process.

As early as possible following the acute event, the patient's physician must assess recovery from infarction and determine what the patient can do now and in the future. These decisions involve a full evaluation of the cardiovascular system, including treadmill testing. Development of an appropriate exercise conditioning program, proper weight, control of blood pressure and the elimination of cigarette smoking are well accepted measures that lower the likelihood of recurrence and enhance the capability for performance. Beyond these well recognized adjuncts, the study of lifestyle involves knowledge of the personal and professional setting and an individualization of the patient's cardiovascular capability in concert with his personal and professional goals.

There is no greater opportunity to successfully modify the behavior of an individual than when his full attention is drawn to an inappropriate lifestyle by a major catastrophic event such as an acute myocardial infarction (see Chapter 5). The physician and nursing staff have the full attention of the patient at this time and can help the patient to achieve a more healthful lifestyle.

I frequently remind myself that a major role of the physician is that of a teacher, and that each patient must be viewed as a student to be graduated with the maximum portfolio of self-care information. Some of the methods available for helping the patient learn to live more healthfully are: establish priorities, identify realistic goals, modify excessive type A behavior, reduce the number of life changes, learn to say no, group or individual therapy, relaxation or meditative techniques, aerobic exercise, and beta adrenergic blockade.[5]

It is unlikely that a patient will adhere to a rehabilitation program if he has had technical intervention without a comprehensive lifestyle assessment. To encourage adherence, behavior modification should be goal oriented with the priorities for modification being selected from the patient's list of risks. Only the two or three most important risks should be chosen from what may well be an overwhelming list. As one adjustment is successfully made, another can be implemented. As one moves down the priority list, management becomes more a matter of fine tuning that major overhaul. One must guard against unbridled zeal for correcting the entire disaster in one massive sweep.

LEISURE

Another dimension of lifestyle which is frequently overlooked in rehabilitation planning is the use of leisure time. One of the greatest misconceptions with regard to the reduction of emotional stress and the "recharging of our psychological batteries" is the modern concept of leisure. The fact that leisure is a major goal of American life is readily apparent in the fact that we spend approximately 20 billion dollars more on leisure than we do on national defense.[6] In a sense, we have converted ourselves from a war economy to a toy economy. Leisure items include everything from motorhomes, motorcycles, electric guitars and airline tickets to swimming pools, tennis courts, pool tables, and belly dancing paraphernalia.

Part of the problem is in the real definition of leisure. According to Dahl,[7] most people think of leisure as free time, that is, time free from work, responsibility, or anything important or significant in their lives. Consequently, it is time to be wasted or time to be "killed". Others think of leisure in terms of getting away from it all, time to be taken out of circulation from the home, from the community, from other people and certainly from any kind of serious engagement with life. Others enjoy experiencing exotic, thrilling and sometimes even violent activities. To still others, it has the general context of personal comforts, conveniences and is identified with the softness and the cushioning of life without discomfort, distraction or inconvenience. We particularly enjoy the nonparticipation in sports ranging from Olga Korbut to Evel Knievel.

For many, however, the stultifying monotony of an occupation or the persistent frustrations of the business or professional struggle may bring about the displacement of achievement goals from business to leisure. Perhaps competition on the tennis court will be more successful than competition in the corporation, and sometimes leadership can be expressed better in social activities than in a frustrating professional setting. For some, this is an essential and healthy psychological adjustment, especially when the leisure is appropriate and balances individual needs with responsibilities. For others, it is an expensive, discouraging, demoralizing detraction which further enhances the feeling of individual loss. Here again, the role of the physician in this setting is to identify which of these two varieties of leisure is appropriate and in balance with his patient's individual needs.

All too frequently, questions related to vacationing are inadvertently omitted. It is sometimes discovered by the physician that the patient never or rarely takes a vacation. For the coronary prone individual, the family vacation may take on a remarkable and frenetic pace. More frequently, it is a four-wheeled family stress test. Distances to be traveled are often far greater than time and the modern speed limits will permit, requiring the addition of electronic devices ranging from citizens band receivers to radar detectors which are generally one microwave step ahead of the local Highway Patrol and two steps beyond reason. It is this type of vacation which I classify as the "we seen it" vacation. The end product of such vacations is an intense exposure to the shortcomings of a variety of factors ranging from one's siblings to one's parents, and certainly not excluding the human bladder. Reflections, should amnesia fail to be an appropriate opiate, consist of a series of blurred photographs of historical markers taken in motion from the family Ford. This brings to mind the necessity for Dramamine® and points out the need for a real vacation following the so-called "we seen it" vacation.

Another side effect of vacations for some is post-vacation depression resulting from unmet expectations and feelings of loss upon returning to the real world from a fantasy world vacation. Any vacation should minimize harassment, time urgency, goal orientation and dehumanization, and maximize human interaction, refreshment and perspective. The family physician's unique opportunity and insight prepares him to provide the best guidance and common sense approaches to these contemporary situations.

Finally, we must remember that active, productive industrious bread winners must be allowed the luxury of dissipating some of their earnings in a way that makes sense and is important only to the spender. A variety of hobbies, equipment and expensive habits abound in our marketplace. These unique expenditures, whether in time or money, may appear senseless, bizarre and wasteful (especially to the spouse). Yet it is the ability to spend time or money on one's fantasy that may make the effort and responsibility of wage earning, parenthood, and marriage a lighter and more acceptable burden or challenge. The happiest of adults retain a little of the child within.

PREVENTION

One of the major problems with prevention of coronary heart disease is the inability to select the individual at risk from the general population or epidemiologic statistics. Another problem with prevention is that the cause of coronary heart disease is multifactorial and not well understood. It is, of course, extremely difficult for anyone to know whether he has prevented a disaster. Medical practice and its rewards function on a more visible and justifiable crisis-oriented basis. Prevention, on the other hand, is often viewed as a cult of dogmatic Psalm-singing Calvinists espousing a lifestyle of the chosen few. Whatever the view, until the pathophysiology is better known, sweeping approaches to prevention represent premature and often misdirected enthusiasm. Today, optimal and prudent health suggestions remain empiric and should, therefore, be made cautiously.

There are many attempts to approach the problem of prevention. Russia, Czechoslovakia, East and West Germany, Switzerland, Austria, Australia, and Sweden all have preventive and rehabilitative reconditioning centers.[8] Each has its own approach, aura, cult, scientific methodology or admixture. Each is aimed at the elimination of physical inactivity, overeating, smoking, and the reduction of emotional and environmental stresses and tensions. In each, the motivating "carrot before the donkey" is that reconditioning is more economical than training replacements.

At this writing, all such data remains soft, interest remains high, yet value remains unknown. If these centers improve the quality of life, it can be argued that they perform a useful function in a turbulent period of human existence. It can also be argued that they must be doing some good if people are willing to pay for their services. If such programs demonstrate an ability to lengthen life as well, their success is a foregone conclusion.

REFERENCES

1. Mullins, C.B.: Early phases of cardiac rehabilitation following a myocardial infarction. Medical Grand Rounds, Parkland Memorial Hospital, Dallas, Texas, November 11, 1976.
2. Cassem, N.H., and Hackett, T.P.: Psychiatric consultation in a coronary care unit. *Ann. Intern. Med.* **75**:9-14, 1971.
3. Klein, R.F., Kliner, V.A., Zipes, D.P., et al: Transfer from a coronary care unit. *Arch. Intern. Med.* **122**:104-108, 1968.

4. Wenger, N.K.: *Coronary Care: Rehabilitation After Myocardial Infarction.* New York: American Heart Association, 1973.
5. Eliot, R.S., and Forker, A.D.: Emotional stress and cardiac disease. *J.A.M.A.* **236**:2325-2326, 1976.
6. Dahl, G.: Personal communication. 1976.
7. Dahl, G.: *Work, Play, and Worship in a Leisure-oriented Society.* Minneapolis: Augsburg Publishing House, 1972.
8. Raab, W.: Preventive myocardiology—proposals for social action. In L. Levi (Ed.): *Society, Stress and Disease,* Volume 1. London: Oxford University Press, 1971, pp. 389-394.

INDEX